Ageless Revolution

...some of the testimonials of Dr. Michael Aziz's patients who followed *The Ageless Revolution* recommendations.

"This anti-aging program is unlike any other program on the market. It is very comprehensive. It targets all ten hallmarks of aging. I absolutely love it."
—Mary S.

"In ten months, I went from 240 pounds to 155 pounds.
I gained my figure back!"
—Sally M.

"I suffered from diabetes, and The Ageless Revolution
helped me to get off all my diabetes medications."
—Brendan B.

"I suffered from high blood pressure for a few years, and I was able to get off the meds. A plan that works better than blood pressure pills is simply magic."
—Kelly C.

"I lost thirty-five pounds in five months, and I am still losing. Amazing!"
—Michael S.

"As a woman in menopause, I got off the dangerous synthetic hormones and started on bioidentical hormones. I got my vitality and energy back."
—Meghan B.

"Dr. Michael Aziz knocks it out of the park with this revolutionary plan."
—Collin L.

"I am a man in his sixties and want to look my absolute best.
The Ageless Revolution helped me achieve that."
—Arthur M.

"At age fifty-four, I feel like I am twenty."
—Tonie L.

"As a senior citizen, I need to know everything new in the anti-aging arena.
Dr. Michael Aziz was my guide."
—Collin A.

THE SCIENTIFIC, BOMBSHELL PLAN THAT TARGETS CELLS AND
DNA TO REVERSE BIOLOGICAL AGE BY UP TO 20 YEARS

The
Ageless
Revolution

10 Hallmarks of Aging
That Hold the Secret
to Defeating Disease,
Reversing Age,
Looking Younger,
and Living Longer

Michael Aziz, MD
Bestselling Author of *The Perfect 10 Diet*

Health Communications, Inc.
Boca Raton, Florida

www.hcibooks.com

This book contains the opinions of the author. This publication provides accurate and authoritative information regarding the subject matter covered. It is sold with the understanding that the publisher is not engaged in rendering legal, medical, or other professional services. If legal advice or other expert assistance is required, the services of a competent professional person should be sought. The advice offered in this book is based on Dr. Michael Aziz's experience successfully treating thousands of patients over the years. The information in this book should not be used as a substitute for your physician's advice on diet, exercise, supplements, medications, procedures, peptides, or hormone replacement.

Readers are advised to consult with their own doctors regarding the treatment of their specific medical problems. Neither the publisher nor the author takes any responsibility for any consequences from any advice, treatment, supplements, hormones, medications, peptides, or procedures to any person reading the information in this book. Many of *The Ageless Revolution* recommendations are not appropriate for people with certain medical conditions, circulation issues, patients with hypoglycemia, pregnant women, and nursing mothers. All brand names and product names used in this book are trademarks, registered trademarks, or trade names of their respective holders.

Library of Congress Cataloging-in-Publication Data
is available through the Library of Congress

© 2025 Michael Aziz, MD

ISBN-13: 978-07573-2514-4 (Paperback)
ISBN-10: 07573-2514-9 (Paperback)
ISBN-13: 978-07573-2515-1 (ePub)
ISBN-10: 07573-2515-7 (ePub)

Publisher: Health Communications, Inc.
301 Crawford Boulevard, Suite 200
Boca Raton, FL 33432-3762

Cover, interior design, and formatting by Larissa Hise Henoch

*Dedicated to all the
visionaries, physicians, and scientists
who made this book a reality*

Contents

Preface

I've been a practicing physician for more than two decades. I trained as a traditional doctor and started a private practice in New York City in 1998. But after a few years in practice, I had a feeling that I was not helping people reach their optimal health goals. Nowadays, people have so many health issues and diseases that it is almost impossible to cover all of them in a short fifteen-minute visit. Seeing twenty-five to thirty patients a day is now the norm in most practices in the United States.

I had this illusion that after fifteen years of medical school and residency training that I'd be able to make a dramatic difference in people's lives. But in reality, many illnesses require more than meds to improve. This requires a lot of time, and counseling, which is impossible to accomplish in our broken and failed medical system.

I was able to help many patients, but it was difficult to make a real impact when everything in the world was working against my efforts. Health misinformation, antiquated dietary guidelines, patients' unhealthy lifestyles, and the fragmentation of the practice of medicine between different physicians were all roadblocks. I grew restless. I questioned my decision to become a doctor. Why did I spend fifteen of the best years of my life studying when I didn't feel I could really make a huge impact on my patients' lives? My gut told me that the key to fixing underlying health issues was to address the underlying problem or go for the root cause of disease.

Since I was fourteen years old, I'd dreamed of becoming a doctor that helps people, and nothing would deter me from my path. So I made a big decision to become a student in my thirties after I thought I was done with all the training. I joined the American Academy of Anti-Aging Medicine to train in functional medicine.

Functional medicine is about treating the root cause of disease, and not placing a bandage on the underlying cause. Every few weeks, on weekends, I would travel to attend a medical conference. I was a student again at the age of thirty-five, but finally, I could see the light at the end of the tunnel. Yes, there is indeed a different way to practice medicine. A much better way.

In time, I had enough knowledge to turn the tables. I became a speaker and began to lecture doctors in the United States and abroad on new research and information. Most importantly, I changed how I treated my patients. They began to see progress, and their health greatly improved.

I wanted to share my newly found knowledge with the public, too, so I decided to write a book. I published *The Perfect 10 Diet* in 2010. In turn, I was featured on many national television shows and in magazines. The book became a national bestseller and was translated into several foreign languages. My life took a new direction that I never envisioned or thought would be possible.

Patients from around the world now seek my medical services. In this book, I will share my personal story and anti-aging knowledge with you, and tell you that there is a different path for you toward health and wellness. There is a new way to age. We can change the trajectory of our health in the United States. In this book you'll find a straightforward, doable plan to age gracefully and possibly live longer. Welcome aboard. Welcome to *The Ageless Revolution*.

Introduction

Life would be infinitely happier if we could only be born at the age of eighty and gradually approach eighteen.
—Mark Twain

IF someone asked you, "Do you want to live past eighty or ninety?" what would your answer be? For most people, it would be a resounding "No." The frailty, illnesses, and loss of mobility that come with advanced age are not appealing.

But what if there is a way to live a longer life disease free, with a sharp mind, vitality, and energy, by reversing your age by a few years or even a few decades? Would your answer still be no? What if Mark Twain's quote above could become a reality?

At one time or another, we've all imagined what it would be like to be young again: when energy, good health, brainpower, and excitement about life filled us with joy. Back then, we took that youth and vitality for granted, and we also lacked the wisdom to appreciate it. As we mature into our forties, fifties, sixties, and even seventies and beyond, we have the experience and wisdom that come with advanced age, but youth and vitality fade, and we feel old.

The Good News About Aging

It's important to keep in mind that our bodies have not failed us. We've just failed to optimize all that the body has to offer. At almost any age, the body still has the means and mechanisms to reboot, reprogram, and reset. All we need to do is find the reset button.

That is what this book is all about: finding the reset button and changing your genetic destiny to revitalize all your cells and organs and become ageless at any age. Call *The Ageless Revolution* your new prescription for youth and vitality.

The Ageless Revolution: An Inside-Out Approach

The Ageless Revolution is a twenty-first-century approach to health and wellness with a focus on disease prevention and cell rejuvenation. It targets the cells. As a result, this plan targets the whole body and organs from the inside out. That's because directly targeting biological aging has many advantages over the traditional one-disease-at-a-time approach. At the present time, living longer, disease free, becomes within your reach.

What Science Tells Us

Today, scientists are actively working to understand the complex process of human aging and developing drugs to slow it down or even reverse it. How far can they go to stretch the human lifespan? Between 1900 and 2020, human life expectancy doubled to 73.4 years. Not bad.

But there was also a remarkable and staggering cost: there was a dramatic rise in chronic and age-related degenerative diseases including heart disease, cancer, type 2 diabetes, arthritis, and Alzheimer's disease.

The good news is that human biology can be optimized. This book teaches you the tools to do just that. You will learn how to get healthy, stay healthy, and enjoy a long, vibrant life.

The Ageless Revolution: Healthy Cells and Longer Life

The Ageless Revolution is all about understanding your body at the cellular level. What you eat, what you do, how the environment and supplements affect you and your cells. Once you understand this, it's easier to appreciate all that your body does for you, and to take better care of it.

Together, we'll work as a team so you can reap the rewards of optimal health and vitality, and add years and even decades to your life. Sound good? I'll bet it does, since you picked up this book. So get ready to embark on an exciting journey with my breakthrough, bombshell, and revolutionary plan. Knowledge *is* power.

I will not lie to you, it will take work, but that's true with anything worthwhile. This includes our relationships, careers or jobs, goals, and dreams. It's no different when it comes to great health. You just need a specific clear plan, consistent attention, and effort, but I promise to make this new, revolutionary way to age easy, doable, and, most importantly, affordable.

Why *The Ageless Revolution* Is Different from Other Anti-Aging Books

The Ageless Revolution is very comprehensive. It is unlike other anti-aging books that cover only diet, exercise, or just futuristic treatments. *The Ageless Revolution* is a step-by-step guide to slowing, and even reversing, aging by directly targeting your cells and DNA.

Think of *The Ageless Revolution* as an inside-out plan to achieve and maintain excellent health. By targeting the cells, a new concept, with all available options and treatments, you can begin to reclaim the energy and vitality that you thought you had lost forever. The message of this book is simple: there is a new way to age.

Why I Wrote *The Ageless Revolution*

Did you know that approximately 95 percent of adults ages sixty and older have at least once chronic condition, while nearly 80 percent have two or more? More troubling news, 68 percent of young adults in the United States have at least two chronic illnesses. With these kinds of odds, you might wonder whether there's anything you can do to prevent the onset of a chronic illness. As a physician, I deal with these chronic illnesses every single day. High blood pressure, high cholesterol, type 2 diabetes, fatigue, and weight gain are some of the diseases that take a toll on the quality of life and lifespan.

Since aging is the most important risk factor for developing these diseases, aging must be targeted head-on. I believe that we can sidestep these types of conditions and diseases by practicing preventive medicine at the cellular level. It is a new concept to deal with aging as a disease that robs us of our health.

Yes, I'm an internist and primary care doctor. But I'm also an integrative and functional medicine physician. This means that I treat the whole person and a disease's root cause rather than a symptom or ailment. You can call *The Ageless Revolution* preventive medicine 3.0 of the twenty-first century.

Getting Old Can Happen at a Young Age

You may be thinking, "I'm too young to read *The Ageless Revolution*." That's not true. There is a worrisome trend happening right now in the United States. Age-related diseases are appearing now in younger people. At present, I see so many young people with obesity, type 2 diabetes, low testosterone, irregular periods, early menopause, arthritis, and the list just goes on and on. Age-related diseases are now affecting the young and old. So, if you want to age gracefully, you need to start young. In fact, the younger you start, the better off your health will be as you get older. For this reason, this book is for everyone, young or old, healthy or suffering from a chronic illness. It is never too early or too late to start. In fact, premature aging can even start in the womb because of the lifestyle choices moms make when they are pregnant. Our mothers' wombs are no longer even safe. Babies at birth now test positive for more than 180 toxins!

Getting Old at a Young Age

Smoking, drugs, poor sleep, stress, or an illness can all speed aging. I learned this important fact during my residency when I was treating HIV-positive patients. The HIV epidemic was just starting, and hospital wards were full of AIDS patients: gay men, hemophiliacs, intravenous drug users, even children and babies.

In the early 1990s, no HIV drugs were available to treat patients, except for a single drug called Zidovudine or AZT. There was one AIDS patient I met during my residency that I will never forget. At the young age of twenty-seven, she was admitted to the hospital where I trained, with an opportunistic infection. Most of us with a healthy immune system do not get sick from these non-harmful organisms. Opportunistic infections, however, are deadly to anyone with a compromised immune system, such as those living with AIDS.

This personable and vibrant young woman informed me that she contracted HIV by having unprotected sex with an older boyfriend. I do not know why she volunteered to tell me this information. Maybe it was her way of avoiding the stigma of me labeling her as a drug user. In those early days, HIV infection was a stigma, sadly, even among medical professionals. I told her that as a doctor, I was not there to judge her. I did not care how she contracted the HIV virus, whether it was unprotected sex, drugs, or a blood transfusion; I was only there to treat her and help her. Happily, she was successfully treated and discharged from the hospital.

But just two months later, she was admitted to my ward again with another opportunistic infection. I happened to be on call that night. By this time, she had been reduced to an unrecognizable, skeletal woman with hollow eyes. She was just skin and bones.

This beautiful patient had aged decades in just a few weeks. Emotionally, I'm a very strong person, but looking at her broke my heart into a million pieces, and I began to cry inconsolably outside her room.

My colleagues, the doctors and nurses, saw me sobbing in the hospital corridor and thought she was a friend or family member. Of course, it's very unprofessional to see a doctor crying. I explained to them that she was a total stranger, but it was impossible for me to be unaffected or feel untouched by such severe human suffering. I prayed for her and hoped that I'd never see such human torment again. AIDS aged this patient decades in just two months. Yes, aging can happen to anyone, even at a young age. That is why *The Ageless Revolution* is for everyone, young and old.

My Journey to *The Ageless Revolution* Book

In late 2019, the Covid-19 pandemic spread throughout the whole world. New York City, where I lived and practiced, became the epicenter of the pandemic in the United States. I was horrified and reminded of the pain and suffering I'd seen in the 1990s with HIV-positive and AIDS patients. Again, Covid-19 made people die, and this time, alone, without their loved ones at their bedside.

The only thing we knew about Covid-19 then was that it was killing older people faster than any other demographic. Aging accelerates the risk of all chronic illnesses: heart disease, cancer, type 2 diabetes, and infections—including Covid-19. But there was something alarming; there were also many young people who got severely sick, suffered more than older people, and died quickly.

The reality is those young folks were old from the inside. They had youthful looks, but their immune system was too weak, just like older people. Why was the immune system of those young people weak to begin with? Why were they so sick and dying at a young age while many older people survived?

Oprah calls it her "aha moment," and I would say this observation made me have my own aha moment when I said to myself, *"Oh my God, those young folks are old on the inside."* My experience in treating both HIV and Covid-19 patients changed my perspective and my focus as a doctor. In turn,

I decided to channel my efforts toward confronting the aging process full force with a variety of weapons. My research, and treating my own patients, inspired me to write *The Ageless Revolution,* starting in 2020. I practice many of the things I preach here, and I need to share my medical knowledge with the public *now.* It would be selfish to keep all my information to myself. The idea to write *The Ageless Revolution* was born.

The pandemic spurred me to refocus my thoughts on all aspects of cellular aging and the science behind why we get old. I wanted to know why both young and old patients were susceptible to dying from Covid-19. I wanted to help sick people get well and help everyone stay healthy for life. We all deserve to live long, healthy, fruitful, and enjoyable lives. We all deserve the opportunity to be as robust as possible for as long as possible and know that we lived well. To do this, I wanted to create a new, revolutionary, bombshell plan.

How Long Can We Live?

Writing a book that challenges the inevitable—aging and death—is not an easy task. You may wonder whether slowing aging is even a possibility! Are we just kicking the can down the road? Well, kicking the can down the road, if it means staying more vibrant and healthier for life, should be everyone's goal. What's so wrong with that! We all want to live longer and be healthy at an older age.

Humans throughout history have searched for the fountain of youth and other ways to slow down aging. Often their methods failed or turned out to be an illusion. But can a human lifespan reach 120 or 125 years? The record holder is Jeanne Calment (1875–1997) from France, who died at 122 years and 164 days old. The strange thing is, she was at one time a smoker, and she continued to smoke until she was 117! The second title holder for longevity is Kane Tanaka, from Japan, who lived until she was 119 years and 107 days old.

There is no doubt that these women were exceptional. Why? How? What did they do to live such long lives? Genes? Lifestyles? Luck? What about the rest of us? How do we become a healthy centenarian or perhaps just reach ninety while still being in good health! No wonder, investors have poured billions into improving longevity, but until relatively recently, there was little progress. Few people in industrialized Western nations reached ninety, let alone did so in vibrant health.

The Ageless Revolution: The Ten Hallmarks of Aging

In 2013, there was a major breakthrough in the world of anti-aging. A landmark paper conceptualized nine hallmarks of aging and their under-lying mechanisms. I added one more hallmark of aging in this book—which is gut health. For me, the ten hallmarks of aging had to be targeted and con-quered. If I found solutions, I solved the puzzle. To my surprise, there were many solutions.

In a nutshell, this book is truly revolutionary because it targets all the ten hallmarks of aging, the malfunctions in our cells, mitochondria, and DNA with those available solutions. It took a lot of work, but it is all gathered in one book.

Today, we can slow down the programmable cell death embedded in our genes. If you think this is science fiction, think again. Think of how people reacted when the Wright brothers flew the first plane in 1903. Now com-mercial flights take us anywhere in the world. Think of how people reacted when Neil Armstrong was the first man to land on the moon in 1969. Now spaceships have reached Pluto and beyond.

We can now target cells and address genetic malfunctions that contribute to aging. Every day we are learning new ways to slow aging. In 2022, three more hallmarks of aging were added. This book will also feature these ad-ditional hallmarks of aging and how to treat them for improved health and wellness and vitality.

The Ageless Revolution: What You'll Learn

In this book I'll share all the breakthroughs and innovations in the last decade that can slow down aging at the cellular level. Believe me, the fountain of youth is not far away. This plan may not enable everyone to live forever, but I'm confident it can improve longevity for many people.

The Ageless Revolution: A New Concept to Fight Aging as a Disease

I won't lie to you; it will take some time to achieve everything that I will share with you. But I believe the quest to fight aging as a disease should be a must for everyone, and the time to do it is *now*. Covid-19 was the test we all took and failed. Take a look around and see how sick we are as a society with all the chronic illnesses plaguing us. So, what are you waiting for? What is stopping you from achieving great health? There may be a moment in your life when you decide it is time to act and get healthier. It could be a New Year's resolution to lose weight. Or it could be a life-changing event like a serious illness that motivated you to pick up this book at your local bookstore or library. Whatever the reason, I am glad you are here.

Aging Well: We Can Do Better

Deciding to adopt healthy habits like quitting smoking, eating nutritious food, or exercising are all good ways to improve our health. But it's not enough. Aging is a mortal enemy. Aging is working against us. Aging sabotages us in so many ways. It damages our cell walls, DNA, and mitochondria. It causes osteoporosis and fractures. Aging changes our skin and appearance.

Nowadays, we are living longer, but not necessarily healthier. We are living with more diseases. Modern medicine failed us by not addressing *aging* as a separate entity or a disease that predisposes us to all these other illnesses. I think of *aging* as a *syndrome* that puts us at risk for several age-related diseases.

The Ageless Revolution Is a Different Approach to Health

It is okay to get older, but it is not okay to get sick. Is there a different path and approach? If there is, why hasn't your doctor told you about it? Maybe he or she is not aware of the ten hallmarks of aging that will be discussed in this book. Maybe he or she is not aware of the natural solutions that can help fight aging or new medications that can protect the cells.

There are plants that have the healing potential to save the world from devastating age-related illnesses. There are supplements that can slow down aging and even reverse it, and we are just starting to learn about them. Many of those supplements target the ten hallmarks of aging. In *The Ageless Revolution*, I will open this treasure chest for you to explore what you can do to change and save your life now.

I've done all the homework for you. I've read tons of research and attended countless lectures to make this book a reality. All you have to do is read or listen to what I have to say. Take in as much as you can. Implement as much information as you can. It is worth the effort. It is your life.

This book will cover heart disease, cancer, type 2 diabetes, obesity, insomnia, fatigue, Alzheimer's disease, autoimmune diseases, skin health, and much, much more. So, if you are looking for a plan to fight all the age-related diseases in a new way that has not been done before, welcome aboard!

The Six Parts of *The Ageless Revolution*

In **Part I, The Science Behind Aging,** I will share with you why we age and tell you about centenarians from around the world. You'll learn about the ten hallmarks of aging, and how to change your genetic destiny.

Part II, Getting Ready to Start *The Ageless Revolution*, will help you get rid of unhealthy habits and carcinogens that are sabotaging your health and longevity. You'll learn about the danger of popular diets: low-fat, low-carb, keto, and other weight-loss programs on hormones and overall health. This section addresses how those very popular concepts negatively affect the ten hallmarks of aging, and in turn, can affect longevity.

Long life is within reach. In **Part III, *The Ageless Revolution* Plan: Principles of the Ageless Diet, Superfoods, Spices, and Longevity,** I will discuss how a healthy, natural, balanced diet has the most impact on longevity. You will understand the principles of a balanced diet, as well as the anti-aging superfoods and spices that will help you live healthier and longer.

Now you are ready! **Part IV, *The Ageless Revolution*,** really gets the program started. I will show you how to turn back the clock with intermittent fasting, and how to do it painlessly. I will discuss the types of exercise you should do for maximum impact on longevity. I will explain which supplements target your cells, mitochondria, and DNA to have the greatest impact on the ten hallmarks of aging. I will also discuss something called *hormetic* stress. It is a type of stress that can fight aging on the cellular level.

Part V, Taking *The Ageless Revolution* to the Next Level with Professional Help. Doctors do not treat aging as a disease. In this section, I take *The Ageless Revolution* to your doctor's office. You'll need a health-care practitioner as a partner for this section. It is the extra steps you need to boost what you already have learned from this book. You will learn how bioidentical hormones can help turn back the clock and how some medications can help you live healthier and longer. I will discuss the latest advances in anti-aging medicine. I'll also explain why we all need a new, innovative approach to our medical care. The model of having a yearly physical is antiquated. You will also learn how to find the right doctor.

Part VI, Embrace the Ageless Life, will summarize *The Ageless Revolution* by condensing all the information together and discussing what it means to have meaning in your life. There is a connection between your brain and your body organs, so it is essential to have a meaningful purpose. A purpose brings joy to your life and enables you to become genuinely ageless.

In the **Appendix,** you will find a detailed **list of foods** and **food plans** to consider while following this new path and easy-to-use **recipes** that add variety to your diet while following *The Ageless Revolution*. In the twenty-first century, manipulating your cells for optimal health and longevity is a reality and within reach. However, it takes much more than eating clean and including exercise in your life for maximum impact. *The Ageless Revolution* will help you learn about and use breakthrough innovations to change your life. You can do it, and you can start right *now*. I will show you what is going on *inside* your body. You will be amazed at the intricate and intelligent mechanisms in your body. You will learn how your body functions, even on a molecular level. You will become aware of just how much you influence the hardworking elements of your body, and how you can slow down aging or even reverse it. This is truly the ultimate ageless revolution. Ready? Let's get started.

PART I

The Science Behind Aging

CHAPTER 1

There Is a New to Way to Age

Aging is not lost youth but a new stage
of opportunity and strength.
—Betty Friedan

Before we get started, let me ask one question, "How do you envision yourself at an old age?" So, take a moment to imagine yourself at an
older, a much older age. Whatever your age now, think decades down the
road. This could make you sixty, seventy, or eighty years old. What do you
see? And how do you envision yourself? Maybe you envision yourself a little
slower, weaker, with less muscles, loose skin, more wrinkles, and gray hair.
We all have seen our parents and grandparents and how they aged. How does
this make you feel? I bet you are not thrilled. Who would be! Right now,
I'm fitter than I was twenty-five years ago, and I was able to turn my health
around with a few simple measures. So when I asked myself the same question and how I would envision myself at a much older age, I had a different
vision of what I would like to be.

I want to be healthy.

I want to be strong.

I want to be in shape.

I want to have great energy.

I want to be active.

I want to be fast.

I want to have a very sharp brain.

I want to be happy.

I want to be independent.

I still want to look good.

This is my vision, and to achieve it, I know I'll need to work to maintain these health goals. There are no guarantees in life, but if I choose a path that can target my cells and DNA and follow simple steps that have been proven to be beneficial in scientific studies, my dream may become a reality. Maybe I can even affect my longevity to live past eighty and ninety, and still be in great health.

The message of this book is simple: there is a new way to age, and I'm ready to share it all with you. For all the dreamers who picked *The Ageless Revolution*, it will take some work, but I assure you it can be done. You can, in short, be old and young at the same time.

Chronological Age Versus Biological Age

Can you truly reverse your age? Is that even possible? You may have heard the saying: "Age is just a number. It's how you feel that is important." This is so true. Who cares if you are seventy years old, if you are in good health, have no serious illnesses, and are full of energy! Wouldn't you love that?

Your age doesn't matter. As you've seen, the reality today is that many people in their twenties and thirties are in even worse health than older generations due to lifestyle choices such as a poor diet, excess drinking, smoking, and drugs.

What's the difference? Chronological age means how old you are according to your date of birth: how long you have been on this earth. But what really matters is your biological age: How old are you from the inside? How old are your cells and organs?

Biological age is a new concept in medicine. It's a way to tell how your cells have changed over time, influenced by lifestyle, illness, and other factors. Let's take, for example, identical twins. One of the twins smokes, and the other does not. The biological age of the smoker would be older than the nonsmoker. Because of smoking, one twin accelerated his biological age even though both twins have the same chronological age and the same DNA.

So how do we know whether a method or a supplement can reverse or slow down aging? In clinical trials, scientists can't wait decades to confirm whether an anti-aging supplement works or not. Instead, they use a metric that measures the effectiveness of different interventions like supplements: they rely on biomarkers of aging.

The age of your cells can be measured by something called the Horvath test, which is based on DNA methylation levels. This biochemical test measures your biological age, your true age. Developed by scientist Steve Horvath, it can actually tell your age from within. Think of 23 and Me, but instead of telling your ancestry, this test tells your cells' age.

But some body organs may have a different biological age than others. For example, a person may have older-looking skin because of chronic exposure to the sun, but he may have a healthy heart like someone younger thanks to healthy eating. Researchers found that proteins in the blood can be used to track the aging of individual organs.

The Ageless Revolution Is Not a Biohacking Book

Using this knowledge, we can now target aging. You hold the keys to your cells. You have heard of hacking computers, hacking emails, hacking elections, and hacking cell phones, but what about hacking your body and cells?

While it may sound like science fiction, biohacking your body and mind can improve longevity. Biohacks include eating better, exercise, supplements, and red-light therapy.

Over the past few years, investment in anti-aging has come from Google, rich tycoons, and crypto millionaires. These biohackers can go to extremes, which can be harmful, like starvation diets and even getting blood transfusions from younger people to reduce their biological age. Bryan Johnson, a billionaire, launched the Rejuvenation Olympics, an online leaderboard, a biohack rivalry of the rich. The winner is the person who can slow down their biological age or age backward the most. Think of Brad Pitt in *The Curious Case of Benjamin Button,* a science fiction movie from 2008 in which he ages in reverse.

How the 0.0001 Percent Fight Aging?

Bryan Johnson spends $2 million a year on supplements, eats seventy pounds of vegetables a month, and never eats pizza or drinks alcohol. So far, he's been able to reverse his biological age by ten years. Jack Dorsey, the ex-CEO of Twitter, now X, eats once a day to stay younger. Elon Musk wants to chip our brains to secure humanity's future. Jeff Bezos is an investor in Alto Labs, a company that researches biological cell reprogramming. Those rich folks are the 0.0001 percent of the people in the world.

But *The Ageless Revolution* is not about extremes. It's about practical and affordable steps that can slow down aging. *The Ageless Revolution* is the new affordable health revolution for the masses.

Some of you may think of me as another biohacker; I am not. I'm a physician who wants to share the latest anti-aging information and knowledge with you. Do I consider myself a biohacker when I watch my diet or exercise? No, I am just trying to take better care of myself. The recommendations in *The Ageless Revolution* are the extra steps you need to age better now. For this reason, I do not want you to see yourself as a biohacker either. I just want you to age gracefully and be in the best health you can be at any age.

Think of Serena Williams, David Beckham, and Lebron James. Those athletes have committed to being in the best shape possible. They have a strict routine of eating right and exercising. When you're committed to your health, you too can win the game of life, and *The Ageless Revolution* can help you do this.

As I've said, I want to be in the best possible health I can be as I get older. After spending most of my life working nonstop and helping patients, I'd love to have some time in my golden years to enjoy the gift of life and experience the magic of the world.

But I also want to leave this world a better place by sharing my knowledge so people can improve their health. To do this, let's begin by taking a closer look at how life began and how our cells work.

Remember . . .

- Biological age is more important than your chronological age.
- There are tests now to measure the biological age of your organs.
- *The Ageless Revolution* is not a biohacking book, but it can change your body chemistry and slow aging.
- Aging should be managed as a disease.
- It's important to keep an open mind as you read the next pages of the book.

CHAPTER 2

Why Do We Age?

Although no one can go back and make a new start, anyone can start from now and make a brand-new ending.
—**Carl Bard**

Before we get started on this revolutionary and new approach to aging better, you will need to understand what is a cell and what is DNA. So please forgive me here if I take you down memory lane all the way to your primary school while I play the role of your biology teacher.

Billions of years ago, life started on earth in the form of a simple cell. Simple organisms like bacteria showed up first, which evolved to live inside other cells, other multicellular organisms, and within mitochondria. Mitochondria, which are organelles found in the cells of most eukaryotes, are hypothesized to have evolved from unicellular organisms more than a billion years ago; they became the battery of our cells, and they contain their own DNA.

The assembly instructions of an animal body are in its genes, acting like an orchestra controlling other cells. After 540 million years, wormlike animals and an explosion of new life-forms with hard ridges, shells, and spines appeared.

These were followed by vertebrates including amphibians, fish, and reptiles. Vertebrates have negligible to little senescence, which is the process of cell degeneration—the loss of power to divide and grow. As a result, vertebrates die a stochastic—non-aging-related—death.

Think of alligators. Alligators only die because they become too large and cannot find enough food to sustain themselves. The same goes for sharks. There are sharks that are over 300 years old in some parts of the world. In the Galapagos Islands and the Seychelles, there are turtles over 200 years old.

Some 175–180 million years ago, non-senescent vertebrates like reptiles evolved into senescent mammals, which experience aging. Of course, that includes us humans. So what happened? Why do we age?

An Expiration Date Is Encoded in Our DNA

It's unfortunate, but every creature on earth has an expiration date encoded into its DNA. Senescence can be seen as a human genetic misfortune. We lost the genetic lottery. However, in practical terms, the fact that sentient lifespans are limited means there is less competition for space and food for the next generation.

Species also evolve to survive. Evolution works best if we reproduce only for several generations, get old fast, and die. This faulty gene makes us deteriorate, or age, just after three or four decades on earth. But today, humans are living longer, with a preponderance for age-related diseases. A seventy-five-year-old man is small and weak. By contrast, a seventy-five-year-old Greenland shark is robust, strong, and shows no signs of aging. It's actually stronger and larger than a twenty-five-year-old Greenland shark. The evolutionary process has placed a poison pill into our mammalian genes.

What You Need to Know About Cell Structure

A cell is enclosed by a plasma membrane around its cytoplasm. It is a barrier that allows nutrients to enter and waste products to leave. The interior of the cell is organized into specialized compartments called organelles. This includes the nucleus, which contains the genetic information for the cell to grow. Other organelles that are present in the cytoplasm include:

- Mitochondria: The battery of the cells.

- Lysosomes: Digest unwanted materials within the cell.

- Golgi apparatus: Packages proteins and separates enzymes.

- Ribosomes: Site of protein synthesis in the cell.

- Centrosome: Organizes the microtubules and provides a structure to the cell.

- Endoplasmic reticulum: Produces proteins for the cell to function.

CELL STRUCTURE

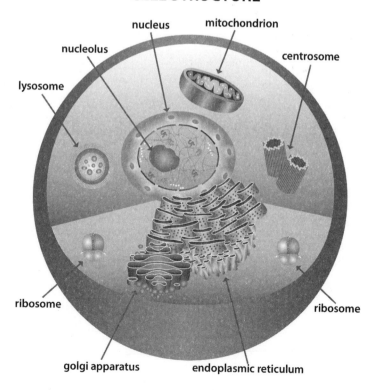

HUMAN DNA

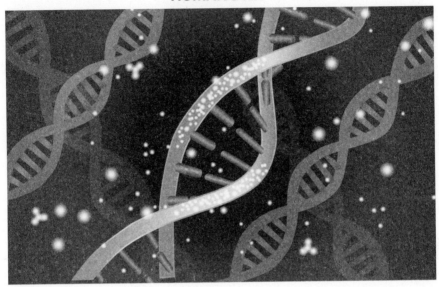

Aging and Cellular Changes

As a result of this genetic misfortune, aging, which is a deterioration of the cells and body organs, happens to all of us. All humans are subject to a chronological age doom. It determines when our cells begin to age and malfunction, and we eventually get old and die. Think of an old cell phone that starts to act up. Maybe the battery doesn't charge, or the screen gets scratched. Eventually, the cell phone doesn't work or dies. It is the same for the cell. The cell membrane gets damaged. The genes get a problem in their code or malfunction. The mitochondria, or the battery of your cell, starts to slow down or die. In turn, diseases happen with advanced age.

Consider this: Smoking increases the risk of getting cancer fivefold. Being over fifty years old increases your cancer risk a hundredfold. At age seventy, it is a thousandfold. Such exponential odds also apply to heart disease, diabetes, and dementia. According to U.S. government statistics, the average human lifespan is eighty-one years for women and seventy-seven for men. It is even a little less after the Covid-19 pandemic.

These lifespans are not bad, especially since according to our DNA, the "healthy and natural" human lifespan should be only about forty years! It's at this time that our cells begin to deteriorate, and diseases arise including high blood pressure, high cholesterol, arthritis, type 2 diabetes, heart disease, and other health issues. Doctor visits become more frequent. It is called aging. While some doctors call aging a disease, I go a step further by calling aging a syndrome. Aging predisposes us to many diseases, including death. We need to address cellular damage in order for us to stay healthier and live longer.

Our Ancient Genetic Code Works Against Us

My patients often complain about these age-related illnesses, "I do not understand, Doc, why do I all of a sudden have high blood pressure and high cholesterol? I exercise and eat right. I am only forty-two!" It has to do with our faulty cells and genes. We are running on an ancient genetic code. Our cells are deteriorating due to the damage to our cell walls and DNA. It is like watching a movie on an old DVD with timeworn scratches versus watching a 4K-definition movie on Netflix or Hulu.

The Myth of Old Age

The notion that we "Die of Old Age'" is a common and misleading myth of modern medicine. We do not die of old age, but rather of cumulative system failures within our bodies. These system and organ failures should not be thought of as inevitable breakdowns but, instead, as reversible elements of aging. Today we now have limitless possibilities to reverse aging at every stage of life. This is the central premise of *The Ageless Revolution*.

Signs of Aging

From our late thirties and early forties, we start to suffer from:

- Cognitive Changes: Slight decreases in cognitive agility and memory recall may begin. Stress and lifestyle factors can impact cognitive health.

- Obesity Risks: Our metabolism slows down. We suffer an increased risk of metabolic syndrome, cardiovascular diseases, and type 2 diabetes. Obesity can lead to an increased risk for many types of cancer.

- Cardiovascular Changes: We start to have clogged arteries, which predisposes us to early heart disease and stroke.

- Autoimmune Risks: Some autoimmune diseases, like rheumatoid arthritis, can start to manifest or worsen.

Defying Nature by Targeting the Cells

Nature has intended, once we're older, that it is time to go and be replaced by a new, younger generation. But we're living longer than ever before. This has its own challenges. Women spend half their adult life in nonreproductive years. What is the quality of their lives without sex hormones? Not good. Although men can reproduce at any age, our health starts to deteriorate in midlife too.

Most doctors focus on treating one chronic illness at a time, but this doesn't help us live longer. To fight diseases of aging, we need to address the body's faulty DNA code. We need to address the cells themselves. We need to treat aging as a separate entity. It is a radical approach that the medical community has yet to embrace.

In the 1900s, life expectancy was around fifty. At this time, people died mostly from a fast death: accidents and infections. Now we are more likely to die a slow death from chronic disease like heart disease, cancer, type 2 diabetes, and neurodegenerative diseases. To achieve longevity, these diseases must be prevented, confronted early on, and conquered.

Modern Life Speeds Aging

There is no doubt that our modern lifestyle is contributing to the development of age-related illnesses. In fact, it's making young people have the same issues as older folks. Our modern lifestyle has accelerated cellular damage and led to these epidemics of age-related diseases happening earlier in life. Think of all those young people who died of Covid-19 because their immune system was too weak, just like old people.

Early humans faced adversity. They had no food for extended periods of time, which meant they were hungrier more often. In fact, the environment was hard for the plants too. There was no massive agriculture. Some of the plants experienced the same harsh conditions, like extreme temperatures and a lack of water, as humans did. As a result, these plants with different colors, such as berries and grapes, had super nutrients. When early humans ate those plants, their benefits passed to them.

Adverse conditions including challenging temperatures from extreme heat to extreme cold made early humans strong and resilient. Today, we prefer to stay at comfortable temperatures. Our food is not only lacking nutrients but also full of toxins and chemicals. Our food now is processed. Our vegetables and fruits are full of pesticides. Animals are also injected with hormones to fatten them up, and we eat these animal products! We snack and eat every three hours. We have little to no time for exercise. Even our carry-on luggage has wheels! This comfort is killing us, accelerating our cells to deteriorate, and ultimately leads to disease and death.

Reversing Your Health as You Age Should Not Be a Dream

New research on animals, like mice, shows that we can slow down cellular aging and improve longevity. But we can also have all the benefits of health that young people enjoy no matter our age. Our minds would be sharp, and Alzheimer's disease would no longer steal treasured memories. We could make clear-eyed decisions, broaden our interests, and be lifelong learners. We could, if we chose to, extend our careers and be productive no matter our age. Our immune systems and physical endurance would be robust, and we'd have far less aches and pains. Heart disease and cancer could be eradicated or become less common. We'd sleep well and enjoy sex no matter our age. We'd have the vitality to enjoy all that life offers us. The possibilities are endless.

From the moment we are born, we begin to age. We all have an expiration date. But it is possible to extend our lifespans to ninety or even one hundred.

I do mean "live," not "exist." I want to be healthy and vital to the very end. No doubt you do too. But is it possible to live to such an advanced age? It is more of a reality than you think—if you're willing to work at it. I don't want to be limited by my age. I assume you don't either.

Over the last century, the human lifespan has slowly extended beyond the range anyone thought possible. Advances in medicine, understanding and controlling infections, better nutrition, and a cornucopia of other medical developments have contributed to our increased lifespans. Still, reaching a one hundred years of age is not the norm.

But in a few areas of the world, many people have cracked the longevity code to live past eighty, ninety, and even one hundred and still be in good health. These areas of the world are called the Blue Zones. What can we learn from them? A lot. You'll see why in the next chapter.

Remember . . .

- Aging is a faulty genetic code in our DNA that makes our cells age, malfunction, and eventually die.
- To target aging, we need to target cellular damage.
- Our modern comfortable lifestyle is accelerating the aging process.
- Our vegetables are now depleted of nutrients and full of pesticides.
- Our food now is mostly man-made and processed.

CHAPTER 3

The Secret of Centenarians Around the World

Every single day, I get up and I say,
I am going to live and not die.
—Tammy Faye Baker

There are places on earth where it's common to find centenarians, which are known as the Blue Zones. First described by a National Geographic explorer and author, Dan Buettner, the five Blue Zones are Ikaria, Greece; Okinawa, Japan; Sardinia, Italy; Nicoya Peninsula, Costa Rica; and in the United States, Loma Linda, California. The name Blue Zones is derived simply from the original survey by scientists, who used a blue pen to map the villages with long-lived populations.

Doctors and ethnographers have found that two major components contribute to those people's health and longevity: diet and genetics. Those folks cracked the longevity code without doing it intentionally. By understanding how and why these people live so long, we can learn more about why we age and how to slow down the aging process.

At first glance, the five Blue Zones do not appear to have too much in common. In fact, they have huge cultural and dietary differences. But it is a constellation of little things that add up to make folks in those areas live past ninety with little heart disease, diabetes, or cancer. One common denominator in the five Blue Zones is a plant-based diet of whole grains, green vegetables, nuts, and beans. A whopping 95 percent of their calories come from plants, and only 5 percent come from animals, foods like beef and dairy. Their diet is not low-fat, low-carb, or keto, which are now in vogue.

Folks in four out of five Blue Zones consume red wine regularly—not in excess. They drink no more than one to two glasses of red wine a day. As for other beverages, they choose water and herbal teas with added oregano, rosemary, and mint. They drink coffee but mostly in the morning.

But their diet is just a part of what adds to their health and longevity. Community is important in Blue Zones and combats loneliness, which can shave eight years off your life.

Three of the five Blue Zones do not have access to industrial roads, which means people walk everywhere, which is one of the best forms of exercise. Let's take a closer look at the Blue Zones and what they can teach us about health and longevity.

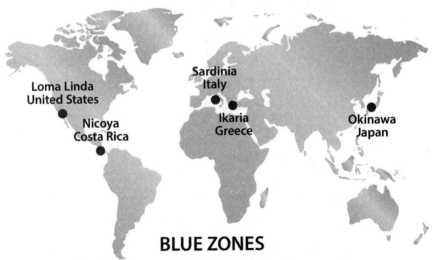

BLUE ZONES

Blue Zones are regions where a higher than ususal
number of people live much longer than average.
There are five Blue Zone areas in the world.

The Five Blue Zones

Ikaria, Greece

Ikaria, also known as Icaria, is a Greek island in the Aegean Sea. Ikarians are almost entirely free of dementia. One in three make it to their nineties. Their food is home-grown, foraged, seasonal, and fresh. In Ikaria, people eat a diet rich in green vegetables, fruits, nuts, and goat milk. Since they are farmers, heavy exercise is inescapable. They are also part-time vegetarians.

In terms of meals, Ikarians typically eat a late breakfast consisting of goat's milk, yogurt, and herbal tea. At lunch, they eat salads made of beans, legumes, and fresh garden vegetables dressed with olive oil. A light dinner consists of bread, olives, vegetables, and wine.

The wine they consume has been prepared the same way for thousands of years with no chemicals. They eat honey that has not been processed. Unprocessed honey has antibacterial activities. Ikarians also have developed a rich herbal tradition, and herbs hold a prominent place in their culture. Meat is eaten about five times a month. They cook, garden, walk, enjoy sex, and socialize into their later years. They are ten times more likely to live past ninety or even a hundred than people in other countries.

Okinawa, Japan

Okinawa's main island is the largest of the Ryukyu Islands located off the coast of Japan. It has the highest concentration of centenarians, 6.5 per 1,000 versus 1.2 per 1,000 in the United States, and is known as the land of immortals.

People in Okinawa eat a vegetable-based diet too, featuring soy, sweet purple potatoes, avocados, shiitake mushrooms, and lots of fish, which can prevent heart disease. The Okinawan diet includes lots of spices and herbs such as turmeric and garlic. They drink lots of green and jasmine tea. Once they eat 80 percent of the food on their plates, they stop before getting too full.

Okinawans do heavy work out in their gardens. They have simple homes with little furniture, so they sit on the floor and then stand up several times a day. This daily routine of getting up and down several times a day helps with their balance as they get older. Okinawans are six to twelve times less likely to suffer from heart disease than people in the United States. They are two to three times less likely to suffer from cancer deaths than in the United States.

Sardinia, Italy

This beautiful island in the middle of the Mediterranean Sea has a ratio of men to women centenarians of one to one versus one to five in the rest of the world. There are ten times more centenarians per capita than in the United States.

The people in Sardinia eat whole wheat bread, garden vegetables, beans, and cheese from grass-fed sheep. Cow, sheep, and goat milk all contain medium-chain triglycerides, or MCTs, which are used for energy and not storage. Of these by far the highest MCT content is present in sheep's milk (about 25%). It contains twice as much lauric acid as goat's milk and three times as much as cow's milk. Sheep's milk also contains much more calcium, phosphorus, iron, and zinc than cow's milk. Red meat is mostly reserved for Sundays or special occasions.

The Sardinians also consume red wine. A whopping 47 percent of their diet comes from whole grains. Yet, the prevalence of obesity in Sardinia is at 0.55 percent! I personally cannot keep the pounds from piling up when I eat just two pieces of bread, so what is the secret of the Sardinians staying in shape? Sardinia has lots of hills, and Sardinians spend lots of time going up and down these hills, on average five miles a day. It is a vigorous form of exercise that burns lots of calories.

Nicoya, Costa Rica

In Nicoya, Costa Rica, where average incomes are among the nation's lowest, the average lifespan is among the world's highest. The big secrets of the Nicoya diet are black beans, corn, squash, papayas, and yams.

People in this sunny area of the world absorb plenty of vitamin D that, in turn, helps absorb calcium. That's because vitamin D is made when our skin is exposed to sunlight. More vitamin D means stronger bones, healthier hearts, and less cancer.

The food here is fresh and locally grown. Their tortillas have refined carbohydrates, but their special preparation of grinding the flour helps release niacin, a B vitamin that plays a big role in health. They prepare and grind their tortillas with their hands, without machines, which also counts as a form of exercise.

Loma Linda, California

Who would ever imagine that there is a Blue Zone right here in the United States! But there is. The Seventh-Day Adventist church in sunny California was founded in the 1840s. The community of 900 church members view health as central to their faith. These members don't smoke or drink caffeinated beverages or alcohol. Loma Linda is the only Blue Zone where alcohol is shunned. They eat vegetables, fruits, nuts, and grains, small amounts of meat, avoid sugar, and exercise regularly. They also have a big social life.

The New Sixth Blue Zone

Some of you may think the five Blue Zones were blessed with some good genes, but they were not. You hold the keys to your own genetic destiny. After a fifteen-year hiatus, Dan Buettner announced that Singapore is the most recent Blue Zone. Singapore was able to become the sixth Blue Zone with policy incentives that encouraged its residents to walk more and to eat healthier food.

In fact, Singapore is an engineered or a manufactured Blue Zone. It is prohibitively expensive to drive a car in Singapore, so walking became a lifestyle for many residents. Singapore's walkways even protect its residents from the sun. Sugar is discouraged. As a result of these government policies, life expectancy has grown in Singapore by thirty years to 83.44 years in 2021, and the number of centenarians doubled in the last decade from 700 to 1,500 in 2020.

Longevity Around the World

In *The Ageless Revolution*, I take you beyond the Blue Zones to discover longevity secrets from around the world.

Monaco

Monaco is number one in the world when it comes to lifespans. The average life expectancy is 93.5 for females, and 85.6 for males. This results in overall health life expectancy of 89.5, which is the lengthiest in the world. Famed for its wealth, glamour, large yachts, and high-stakes gambling, Monaco also gives its citizens a top-notch health-care system, high-quality doctors, near year-round sun, stress-free living, and a healthy Mediterranean diet. Fish, seafood, and red wine, which play a role in longevity, are all staples in their cuisine.

Stress often shortens people's lifespans. Here, high-end living reduces stress, which means that residents are likely to be happy and live much longer. Monegasques are comfortable financially, but the great wealth in Monaco is mostly with foreign expats, so do not be fooled that you need tons of money to live a long life.

Hong Kong

Hong Kong also shares the number one spot in lifespans with Monaco, with a life expectancy at eighty-eight years for women and eighty-two years for men. Hong Kong cuisine has many similarities to Mediterranean cuisine. The Mediterranean diet is linked to longevity since it is rich in vegetables, fruits, beans, olive oil, and an abundance of seafood. Hong Kong's position as both a marine and land gateway to China and other parts of Asia enable greater access to fresh seafood, vegetables, and fruits. Their Asian diet limits oils for cooking. Meat is chopped up into dishes rather than eaten as whole portions. This means smaller portions. Less food means longevity as I will discuss later in this book.

Tai chi, the ancient martial arts practice of self-defense, also improves balance and concentration and is practiced by seniors at public parks all over Hong Kong. Seniors who participate not only can socialize but also improve overall well-being. Both exercise and socialization play an important role in longevity.

South Korea

Moving on to South Korea, women routinely live longer than ninety years on average. Talk about longevity! What is their secret? Compared to women from thirty-four other industrialized nations, South Korean women generally smoke less, weigh less, have lower blood pressure, and see doctors more often because most have health insurance. Their long lifespans of course are related to all those factors, but it may come down to a South Korean dish called kimchi. Kimchi is based on fermented vegetables—usually cabbage—which is high in probiotics and vitamins A and B. Fermented products play a huge role in longevity. Gut health is one of the ten hallmarks of aging.

Longevity in the United States

The average life expectancy in the United States is 78.8 years, well below neighboring Canada (82.3 years) and nearly all other high-income countries. We are ranked at a mediocre number forty-two in longevity in the world and plagued with many age-related diseases, including obesity, diabetes, and high blood pressure. Something is terribly wrong when the richest country in the world, the one that spends the most on health care, is so far behind. With more than a third of all Americans now over the age of fifty, we need a revolution to get us out of the gutter.

Age-Related Diseases Are Plaguing the Western World

But it's not just those who are fifty and older who are experiencing age-related diseases. Today, we are experiencing an even more frightening phenomenon. Aging is happening at a much younger age in the Western world. Insomnia, low testosterone, menstrual irregularities, even cancer are happening much more in both young men and women. ADHD and memory issues in children have increasingly become more common. The young are aging sooner and faster than ever before. This shouldn't be happening. With all the new knowledge you will learn from this book, it is time for us to change our genetic destiny.

What Is Syndrome X and How Does It Affect Longevity?

Forty percent of the United States population is now obese. In the 1960s, an endocrinologist named Gerald Reaven observed that excess weight often goes with poor health. He noticed that heart attacks often happen in patients with high sugar, high triglycerides, as well as elevated blood pressure. In the 1980s, Reaven called this cluster of disorders syndrome X.

Today, syndrome X is called metabolic syndrome. According to recent research, as many as 120 million Americans have at least one of the metabolic syndrome criteria below. If you have three of the six issues below, you may have metabolic syndrome, which can lead to diabetes. Do you have . . .

* Insulin resistance? This means when the cells do not respond to the insulin secreted from the pancreas and the sugar remains elevated in the bloodstream.
* High blood pressure?
* High triglycerides?
* Low HDL cholesterol (good cholesterol)?
* Central adiposity (big waistline—40 inches in men and 35 in women)?
* Elevated fasting sugar level?

If you have one of those points, don't despair, this book will help you turn your health around.

Our Modern Diet

Diabetes is now an epidemic in the Western world. That's because our environment has changed so much faster than our genome. Early humans needed to endure periods of time without food. So our genes enabled us to survive famine. Now in the developed world, we have unlimited access to calories.

When it comes to sugar this can be especially problematic. Too much sugar can lead to insulin resistance. Again, this is when the cells don't respond to insulin, a hormone that allows sugar to enter. As a result, sugar remains elevated in the bloodstream. This is the first step in metabolic syndrome, and it opens the door for all modern diseases that shorten life: heart disease, stroke, diabetes, and Alzheimer's disease. Fast food is now everywhere with an abundance of refined carbohydrates and trans fats in our diet. Trans fats interfere with nutrients going into the cells and all cellular communications, which leads to more insulin resistance.

My Trip to Sardinia

Seventeen years ago, I traveled to Italy and had the chance to spend a few days in Sardinia, one of the five Blue Zones. The island is quite remote and has escaped the "progress" of Western civilization for thousands of years. When I bought some fruit from a local vendor and part-time shepherd, he was curious about where I was from and what I did for a living. When I told him that I am a physician, he remarked that he had never gone to a doctor before. He was a healthy eighty-eight years young. Although I didn't know about the Blue Zones at the time, I now realize the key for his longevity. Eating locally grown food, foraged food, walking up and down the mountains with his sheep, a friendly attitude, and a purpose in life to take care of his family must be his secret.

My Trips to Monaco

I have attended many medical conferences in Monaco over the years, and here too, much of the secret to longevity can be found in lifestyle and the cuisine. Monaco cuisine takes influence from French and Mediterranean cuisine. Bouillabaisse is a rich seafood stew high in omega-3 fatty acids. Ratatouille is a vegetable stew made of eggplant, bell peppers, zucchini, and fresh herbs. The vegetables come fresh from the farms. It is a favorite for locals. Another local dish is socca, a lovely crepe made with chickpea flour. It is also flavored with olive oil and fresh herbs. The Monegasques also cracked the longevity code.

The Blue Zones and Plant-Based Diets

Blue Zone diets are mostly plant-based, unlike the Standard American Diet, which is high in sugar, trans fats, and chemicals. The American diet is also high in red meat and processed foods.

In each of the countries in the Blue Zones, through diet and lifestyles, they have changed their cells, DNA, and destiny. They've cracked the longevity code without knowing it. But you don't have to move to any of the five Blues Zones to enjoy a long, healthy life. In fact, in *The Ageless Revolution* I will bring you longevity secrets from the people all over the world who have lived the longest.

A Patient's Story

Most people tend to go to the doctor when they are sick or only when they need to. That was the case of Molly, one of my patients who had not seen a doctor for years. Molly was a forty-five-year-old woman who walked into my office a year ago with no real complaints. She was simply interested in losing thirty pounds. Her family history was unremarkable; the only red flag was that her father had dementia at seventy. I set up another appointment in a week to follow up on her test results. But there were few things that were alarming about her physical exam. Her sugar was high, indicating she was prediabetic. Her lipoprotein (a), which indicates a high risk of heart disease, was high. Her labs also revealed she had the APOE e4 allele, which is associated with a greater risk for Alzheimer's disease. In circumstances like this, I generally think it is best to get right to the point. Molly was devastated, but the point I tried to make to her was that time was on her side. She was young. It was not only time for her to lose weight but also to address all her other risk factors that predisposed her to three of the worst diseases that face us as at an older age: diabetes, heart disease, and Alzheimer's.

The prevention plan was an aggressive treatment that included a diet low in sugar, controlling her metabolism and sugar abnormalities, increasing her consumption of fish, and reducing alcohol. It appears anaerobic exercise or strength training plays a big role in preventing Alzheimer's disease. It was time for her to take exercise more seriously. Sleep is also a powerful tool in the fight against Alzheimer's disease, and many nights Molly stayed up late.

As she incorporated all my guidance, she started to see results and lost some weight. Optimizing her sex hormones was also on the list as balanced sex hormones can help prevent Alzheimer's disease. After one year, Molly lost all the excess weight, her sugar normalized. Although the genetic factors remain, her risks for developing those three devastating diseases have been greatly reduced.

Remember . . .

- People in the five Blue Zones live longer by eating a plant-based rich diet and having an active lifestyle.
- You can crack the longevity code by changing your DNA with your lifestyle.
- Fermented products play a role in longevity as they play a role in gut health, one of the ten hallmarks of aging.
- Kimchi may be the secret of longevity for South Korean women.
- Red wine plays a role in longevity.
- Stress-free living is linked to longevity as it lowers cortisol, a stress hormone.
- Age-related diseases are now happening in younger generations.

CHAPTER 4

The Ten Hallmarks of Aging

Once you stop learning, you start dying.
—**Albert Einstein**

If people in the Blue Zones cracked the longevity code by targeting cellular deterioration with diet and lifestyle changes, you can do it too. Aging is described as an overall cellular breakdown that leads to impaired function, which in turn leads to death. Aging is the major risk factor for chronic diseases that ruin health and shorten lifespan.

I explained to you functional medicine. It targets the root cause of disease, not the symptoms. So if we examine aging, we need to know why it happens. Why do the cells deteriorate? To solve the puzzle, I had to totally understand what went wrong. To my surprise, for most of the hallmarks, there were many remedies. I only had to assemble this information.

In 2013, a team of researchers attempted to identify and categorize the cellular and molecular hallmarks of aging. They sorted the causes of aging into nine distinct scientific hallmarks that interact with one another and drive the onset of age-related diseases like heart disease, type 2 diabetes, cancer, and Alzheimer's disease. As the cells get damaged, disease happens. This breakthrough research has been cited a thousand times in journals, research studies, and conferences.

Today, there are multiple available therapies, and more are being discovered, that can intervene in the aging process. For each hallmark of aging, you'll learn what to do from lifestyle changes, diet, and supplements to take. Do not get discouraged or overwhelmed by the name of the drugs or supplements. This chapter is only an introduction, so don't make shortcuts to the end of this book. The information shared here is lifesaving and life-changing. Understanding the ten hallmarks of aging, the glitches that are in our DNA and cells, is key to helping you live a longer and healthier life.

The Ten Hallmarks of Aging

1. **Loss of stable cell synthesis of protein.** You need protein of good quality for your cells to work properly. As environmental stresses add up, the mechanisms responsible for proper protein composition in the cells start to decline. In other words, the protein made in the cells is mediocre. Autophagy is the process of destruction of damaged or redundant cellular components occurring within the cell. Misfolded, damaged proteins accumulate, and the proteins inside the cells of your body are no longer of excellent quality. It is these proteins that dictate the health of the entire cell and what cells create.

   Think of those bad proteins as workers in a company who call in sick a lot due to an illness. The other employees in the company must work harder to cover for those who are sick and absent all the time, so eventually, all the employees get tired.

   If one cell is sick because its proteins are out of order, soon all the cells around it will be in trouble too. They will have to work harder to cover for the sick cells that do not do their jobs. When the system goes out of balance, there is an open door for all kinds of illnesses. Keeping the proteins in your cells healthy ensures your entire system is healthy, stable, and youthful.
   Available therapies: Intermittent fasting and a drug called low-dose naltrexone.

2. **Altered cell communications.** Cells need to communicate with one another and sense nutrients for your body to function properly. Think of it this way: If two people are trying to talk to each other on their cell phones but have a poor signal, they will not understand what the other is saying or asking them to do. Then, when they try to do what they think they were told, they will do the wrong thing or nothing at all. Our cells behave just like people do in this regard. Altered cellular communications happen for a variety of issues. Cells need hormones such as insulin and sex hormones to talk. If your hormones are not balanced or healthy, they can't tell your cells what to do to keep you healthy and highly functioning. Metabolism and its by-products damage cell walls via oxidative stress. Think of your cells as a house that needs functioning windows for air and oxygen to come in. If the windows are shut, the people inside the house will not be able to breathe. It is the same for the cells. In turn, nutrients and hormones cannot go in.

   Available therapies: A natural diet, minimization of free radicals, optimization of hormones.

3. **Loss of stem cells.** We were made from sperm and an ovum when our mom and dad came together. In other words, we came from stem cells. Those early cells differentiated to what we are today: brain, muscle, and skin cells. Stem cells can turn into any cell you want them to be. Stem cells are unspecified cells, so they can divide, renew, or become more specialized. After our body and different organs are made, 700,000 stem cells remain in our bodies, mostly in the bone marrow. Those remaining stem cells are used whenever we need them. As we age, we deplete those remaining stem cells, but the stem cells also lose their ability to regenerate. Stem cells are like that old comic book hero Plastic Man. Plastic Man could turn himself into anything. If you need a key to open a door but do not have one, Plastic Man becomes the key. If you need to see something at a distance but do not have binoculars, Plastic Man comes to the rescue. Even though stem cells turn themselves into keys

or binoculars or anything else, they can make themselves into absolutely any kind of cell your body needs to be healthy. Need a few liver cells because there has been some liver damage? No problem. Your stem cells will turn themselves into new liver cells. Stem cells' ability to become whatever kind of tissue or organ you need is what keeps you alive, regenerating, and thriving. By age sixty to seventy, we are out of most of our stem cells. When your stem cells run out, so do you. But don't despair, *The Ageless Revolution* is here now for the rescue.

Available therapies: Consuming certain superfoods such as black tea and dark chocolate can help stem cells stay alive longer, stem cell infusions, a peptide called GHK-copper, and hyperbaric oxygen chambers may help.

4. **Deregulation nutrient sensing.** Cells throughout the body require a constant supply of nutrients to provide energy, and the cells are able to store them. Cells sense these nutrients to adjust sugar levels by using signaling mechanisms. Multiple nutrient-sensing pathways regulate intake to provide just the right amount of nutrition.

The Pathways for Cellular Health

Think of your body as a luxury hotel with four different elevators. Your cells are the hotel's guests. The pathways are the hotel's elevators for the delivery of food. There are four elevators in the hotel that are used to bring food from the various restaurants. A sort of in-room service. There is an elevator for the food from the breakfast restaurant, which supplies mostly carbs. This is the IGF-1 pathway, which stands for insulin and insulin-like growth factor signaling pathway (IIS). It handles carbs. There is an elevator for a steakhouse restaurant, which serves mostly steak or protein. This is the mTOR pathway, which stands for the mammalian target of rapamycin. It handles protein. There is an elevator for a mixed restaurant, which serves a variety of food, both carbs and protein. This is the AMPK pathway, which stands for adenosine monophosphate-activated protein kinase. It handles both carbs and protein. There is also an elevator used only in emergencies when all the restaurants in the hotel are closed. This elevator is only used to make sure the guests are okay and safe when all the hotel restaurants are closed, and no food is around. This is the sirtuins pathway. It works with intermittent fasting.

If three (IGF1, AMPK, and mTOR) of these pathways get used all the time, they start to break down. These pathways are essential for cellular health and must be functioning optimally. Think of it this way: If the hotel's elevators are used all the time to bring food to the guests nonstop, they will break down in no time from overuse, especially when the building gets old. As a result, the hotel's guests will suffer with no food around. The hotel becomes uninhabitable. These pathways slow down and fail as we get older. In turn, aging happens. All these pathways facilitate nutrient transport, and they become less efficient as we age. Excess food activates these pathways the wrong way and can lead to a shorter lifespan. Evidence generated so far strongly suggests that diminished nutrient signaling in some pathways culminates in an extension of a cell's life cycle. Now we understand the longevity of Okinawans in Japan, who stop eating when they are 80 percent full. Excess food leads to a decline in the functional reserve of a cell and expedites aging. In other words, overeating accelerates aging.

Available therapies: Limiting sugar, limiting animal protein. A compound called NAD, caloric restriction, exercise, curcumin, and resveratrol. Two potent activators of AMPK, a pathway in the cells that regulate nutrient sensing, are hesperidin, which comes from citrus fruits, and a plant from Asia called jiaogulan. A drug for diabetes called metformin optimizes the AMPK pathway. One drug that is controversial and acts on the mTOR pathway is called rapamycin. Excess heat, cold, and intermittent fasting also optimize the sirtuins pathway.

5. **Loss of telomeres.** Telomeres are the end caps of chromosomes. The term comes from ancient Greek. Telos means end, and meres means part. As cells divide, the telomeres at the ends of chromosomes get shorter. Telomeres are like plastic caps at the ends of our shoelaces. Without them, our shoelaces would fray and eventually shred and become useless. Our chromosomes are just like shoelaces because they can fray too, but not from walking around and getting caught in an escalator. Chromosomes can fray every time your cells divide. Cell division

is vital, but fraying telomeres are dangerous. Every time a cell divides, the chromosomes divide too, and without telomeres, those chromosomes might not be identical in each of the new cells. That is how mutations happen. Mutations create disease and compromised cells, which create—you guessed it—aging and death. Eventually, the enzyme that adds telomeric repeat sequences, telomerase, gets silenced, and the telomeres are too short for the cells to successfully divide.

Available therapies: A diet high in seafood, a good sex life, a supplement extracted from astragalus root, vitamin D3, selenium together with ubiquinol, and fish oil—all these measures help make your telomeres longer.

TELOMERES

telomeres

chromosome   cell division   telomere
                                                                shortening

Telomeres Shortening with Each Cell Division

6. **Aging cell accumulation.** This is exactly what it sounds like. A cluster of aging, damaged, poorly functioning cells accumulates in an area of the body. These damaged cells could be lurking within our bodies, stalking otherwise healthy cells, and spreading a plague of dysfunction in their wake. For example, say the pancreas has some aging cells. Those aging cells in the pancreas are deeply disruptive and unhelpful to the healthy cells. Those healthy cells around the unhealthy cells start to fail too. Think of it like this: The body is like a car where some older parts are poorly functioning. Those older parts are not only slow, but they also

can damage the whole car performance by slowing down the other functioning parts. As a result, the car breaks down.

This is what happens inside our bodies. Old cells are not productive but also secrete inflammatory chemicals and cytokines that disrupt the young cells from working properly. In time, all the cells in the body start to fail. Those aged cells create chaos, so scientists call them *zombie cells*; Human studies have not been initiated, but when scientists injected mice with drugs that kill those *zombie cells*, they noticed a noticeable improvement in the aging process. The mice were treated with a class of drugs called senolytics (drugs that kill the senescent, or zombie, cells), the mice who got treated were more agile and alert.

Available therapies: Intermittent fasting, a drug called metformin, a drug called rapamycin, curcumin, some supplements such as fisetin, quercetin, and others that will be discussed.

7. **Chromosome instability.** This is the accumulation of damaged DNA. As cells age, the chromosomes become less stable. As repair fails to correct DNA damage, mutations occur. When I was a teenager, I listened to the newest hits on the radio, but I wanted to hear those hits all the time. Back then, there was no Internet or YouTube. A friend of mine would copy these new hits I liked from his brand-new CD to a new blank CD. So now I had the latest hits, but the quality of music was always inferior to my friend's original CD. Guess what would happen if I gave my mediocre-quality CD to someone else to copy? The quality of the sound would be even poorer! Repeat again, and the sound quality will make the next CD copy incomprehensible. And if your CD is scratched, the information embedded cannot be transferred to a new CD at all. If a chromosome that holds all the information about what your body needs is unstable (like a scratched CD), it cannot do its job either. When a chromosome cannot supply the information, the added information is wrong. Guess what happens? Mutations.

Available therapies: Intermittent fasting, a drug called metformin, a molecule called NAD, and a drug called low-dose naltrexone.

8. **Mitochondria dysfunction.** Mitochondria are the batteries of your cells and produce energy, which makes everything in your body run properly. Would your car be able to run without a charged battery? Can your cell phone make a phone call without being charged? Can your body run without mitochondrial energy? No. We need healthy mitochondria for all our cells to work. There is also a relationship between shortened telomeres and mitochondrial dysfunction. Everything in the cell must work. Would you be able to use your cell phone if the glass screen is broken but the battery is charged? Of course not. The same goes for your cells. In other words, if your telomeres are short, the mitochondria or battery of your cells start to fail too.

    Available therapies: Good sleep hygiene, a molecule called NAD, low-dose naltrexone, red light therapy, a supplement called urolithin, and an antioxidant called glutathione.

9. **Epigenetic alteration.** The term *epigenome* is derived from the Greek word *epi*, which means above, and the genome, which is DNA. Epigenetic alteration is what happens when a chemical compound attaches to the genome, or the DNA, in a way so as to tell the cells what to do. Think of your life as a movie. Your cells are the actors and actresses. Your DNA or genome is the movie script. Epigenetic alteration is the movie director. The director can make the movie a success or a failure. The director may make a comedy (happy movie) or a horror movie out of your life. By telling the actors and actresses what to do, the director can also delete scenes by editing the script. The director can also push an actor to act their absolute best so that he or she may win an Oscar. Or the director may even decide to kill the actor in the middle of the movie by flipping the script. The end result can be drastically different depending on what the director wants. After all, a movie directed by Steven Spielberg will be vastly different from a movie directed by

Martin Scorsese. Epigenetic alterations are the good or bad things we do in life. They alter your life. Think of smoking; it leads to cancer. Think of nitrites in processed meats; they have been linked to colon cancer. In fact, colon cancer was the first cancer linked to epigenetic alteration. Our unhealthy habits make our genes act in a bad way and change how our DNA reacts. There are twenty-three pairs of genomes in a human cell. Damage happens over time as cells get exposed to bad environmental factors such as smoking, drinking, and drugs.

Available therapies: Lifestyle changes, a balanced diet, and a drug called metformin.

10. **Gut health.** Although this hallmark was not included in the original nine hallmarks of aging, I added it because I feel gut health is crucial to longevity. Researchers added it in 2022. Inside our gut, there are bacteria that secrete vitamin K2, which supports heart health, and a chemical called urolithin, which helps protect the mitochondria. Gut bacteria also play a role in brain health, weight, and emotions.

Available therapies: A proper diet high in fiber and fermented products; more on gut health in Chapter 13.

The Addition of Three More Hallmarks of Aging in 2022

During the writing of *The Ageless Revolution*, three more hallmarks of aging were added in 2022. Those three additional hallmarks are compromised autophagy, chronic inflammation, and dysbiosis. Compromised autophagy means not only bad proteins, but all other cell parts such as damaged DNA, are not digested. Think of it this way: If your car has a damaged windshield, flat tire, and a broken rear light, what would you do? You need to replace all damaged parts of the car with new ones. Again, we need to get rid only of not old damaged protein but all the damaged parts of the old cells. The other hallmark that was added is chronic inflammation, which happens as we get older. There is an increase in inflammatory markers secreted from the old cells. It is very similar to old cell accumulation. The toxins secreted from the old cells impair the functioning cells. Again, we need to get rid of the old cells. Dysbiosis is really gut health, which I already discussed and added on my own, so I was right to discuss it in *The Ageless Revolution.*

In summary, there are ten hallmarks of aging that we must conquer to fight cellular damage. Now you know why we age and die. Depressed? No need to be. *The Ageless Revolution* is bringing you the latest research information so you can finally do something about it. I have assembled all sorts of weapons for you.

Remember . . .

- There are ten hallmarks of aging:
- Proteins in cells lose their efficiency, become damaged, and bunch up, so cells in the vicinity malfunction.
- Cells lose communication between one another because of hormone imbalance, poor metabolism, and metabolism by-products. Cells then cannot understand one another and cannot do their jobs.
- Stem cells become whatever your body needs—new cells or even tissues. When you exhaust your stem cells, death follows.
- Deregulated nutrient sensing. Cells use four different pathways to detect nutrients. With aging, some of these pathways become less efficient.
- Without their important telomeres, chromosomes cannot divide, or divide incorrectly, and eventually there is no more cell division.
- When cells become damaged or die, they sometimes accumulate and disrupt nearby healthy cells, and all the cells start to fail.
- Chromosomes are in the nucleus of living cells. When DNA is incorrectly repaired or degraded, chromosomes cannot supply correct information to the new cells.
- Mitochondria are the energy source for all the cells throughout the entire body. When this energy in the battery runs out, so do you.
- Epigenetic alteration is the damage done to the genomes by the environment.

- Having healthy gut bacteria is essential for longevity.
- Three additional hallmarks for aging were added in 2022 but are similar to the ten discussed in *The Ageless Revolution.*

CHAPTER 5

You Can Change Your Genetic Destiny

*Every time you are tempted to react in the same old way,
ask if you want to be a prisoner of the past
or a pioneer of the future.*
—Deepak Chopra

Certainly, the idea that you can directly affect your health and longevity through lifestyle and diet is not a new one. Spas and health retreats have been popular all over the world for millennia, all built with one purpose in mind: to get healthy and stay healthy. In 70 AD, the Romans built a spa in Britain around a thermal spring in Bath, which became a health center and a gathering place. For anyone who is up on their Jane Austen books, many of her characters live or visit Bath, not only for the social excitement, but for the health-supporting spring water.

Not to be outdone, Americans quickly caught on to the British craze. In 1815, the first public thermal baths in the United States were founded in Saratoga Springs, New York, with luxury hotels modeled after the Roman revival style. Later, as times passed, more services were offered as spas expanded and reflected the needs and desires of the patrons. Among those services was weight reduction.

In turn, the American diet and wellness industry began its meteoric climb to a national obsession. In 1876, Dr. John Harvey Kellog took over the Western Health Reform Institute in Battle Creek, Michigan, and reinvented it as Battle Creek Sanitarium. Yes, that's the same Dr. Kellogg who branded the famous cereals.

Dr. Kellogg encouraged and administered yogurt enemas, had guests sleep outdoors, and strapped quite a few of his guests into slapping machines for automated pummeling. But not all his methods were that wacky. As an early proponent of the germ theory of disease, Dr. Kellogg was years ahead of his time when it came to the role of intestinal flora in health and disease. He used colon-cleansing enemas and recommended abstinence from tobacco, alcohol, and sexual activity. At that time, syphilis was a disease that shortened people's lives.

Naturally, part of Dr. Kellogg's treatment was focused on nutrition. A quick review of the sanitarium's menu reveals that absolutely no meat was offered, the size of each meal was small, and yogurt was eaten for its probiotic qualities. By the early 1900s, calorie counts accompanied every item on the menu. The health benefits of nuts were of great interest to Dr. Kellogg, who pioneered the creation of meatless meat (back in the headlines again today), using nuts and wheat.

Who knows whether those products would still be eaten today if they had been given better names? Nuttose, Protose, and Nuttolene did not have appetizing or sexy names that appealed to the public beyond Battle Creek. Yet, these meatless meats were around long before Beyond Meat and other faux meats popped up in today's supermarkets. Protose was available until the 1990s, and today the Kellogg company continues its interest in meat-like alternatives. Dr. Kellogg, who died at the ripe old age of ninety-one, did many things right, but his health methods and treatments were often underappreciated in his lifetime.

Unbeknownst to these sanitarium patients who wanted a smaller waist-line, more radiant skin, and a better digestive system, they were also altering their own DNA. More precisely, they were altering the way their bodies interacted with their DNA. That sounds a little like science fiction! Yet altering our DNA through our lifestyle choices, food, and activities is a process scientists, researchers, and doctors advocate today. It is called epigenetics. Epigenetics is the movie director who can make the actors (your cells) shine or die.

Epigenetics

According to the Centers for Disease Control and Prevention (CDC), "Epigenetics is the study of how your behaviors and environment can cause changes that affect the way your genes work. Unlike genetic changes, epigenetic changes are reversible and do not change your DNA sequence, but they can change how your body reads a DNA sequence."

Think of epigenetics as the needle in the vinyl record player. If it is damaged, no good music can be played. Imagine for a moment if Whitney Houston was a total unknown, and for a chance at stardom, she sent a demo of her songs to *The Voice* (pretend it existed in the 1980s.) But there was a major mishap: The producer who played her demo's voice recording to the judges used a vinyl record player with a damaged needle! Whitney Houston sounded so off she was not selected even for the first round of auditions! It was a tragedy. Whitney lost her chance, and the public never heard one of the greatest voices of all time. That shows you how the bad things you do can negatively affect your DNA. Whitney Houston's voice is the same, but the damaged needle ruined her chance for stardom.

Epigenetic Alteration: Making Your DNA Work for You, Not Against You

Epigenetic alteration is the first hallmark of aging we must target. Epigenetic alteration is modification in gene expression; it turns on pro-aging genes and shuts down youthful-promoting genes.

Epigenomes are chemical compounds and proteins that attach to your DNA and then tell your DNA what it should or should not do. In other words, epigenomes are like a bossy fifth grader telling an otherwise unsuspecting third grader what to do during recess. The bossy kid (the epigenome) might tell the third grader (your DNA) to stop hitting another kid over the head with a notebook. That is good! Conversely, the bossy kid might tell the little kid to leave a rubber spider on the teacher's chair. That is not good! In both situations, the third grader is the same person but is being motivated or triggered to behave in a particular way. As a result, the principal bans all third graders from play time.

This is exactly what happens when the epigenome attaches itself to the DNA. It is called DNA methylation. It is "marking" the DNA and leaving a record of the activity so that the same activity can be started up or turned off in the future. In other words, the good and bad things you do affect how your genes will act in the future. Good things like fasting will turn on the repair mechanisms of your DNA, or genome. The cells start to regenerate. Bad things like overeating will turn off your repair mechanisms for your genome. The cells will start to deteriorate. Epigenomes are prompting your DNA, and consequently the cells in your body, to stop aging and repair itself. They're the key to longer lifespans and greater health.

Sirtuins Are the Heroes

When we dive deeper, we find that the real heroes in epigenetics are proteins called *sirtuins*, which exist in every cell in our bodies. Sirtuins are a family of signaling proteins. They include sirtuins that occupy various parts of the cells: SIRT1, SIRT6, and SIRT7 are in the nucleus of the cells; SIRT2 is in the cytoplasm; and SIRT3, SIRT4, and SIRT5 are in the mitochondria.

In 1979, a paper announcing the discovery of a gene regulator was published. It controls the mating and sterility in yeasts. Three more proteins were discovered in the same year and the nomenclature was unified, thus creating a family of SIR (Silent Information Regulator) and proteins. Since then, we have learned that sirtuins are found in most organisms, including plants, bacteria, and animals, and play a key role in promoting an organism's health.

Sirtuins attach themselves to our DNA to tell cells to do fantastic things like live longer, be resistant to disease, and feel more vibrant regardless of age. They are indispensable for DNA repair, controlling inflammation, and antioxidative defense.

So, increasing the sirtuins in your body and finding ways to activate them to do their magnificent work on your DNA is a smart thing to do. Other than ingesting pharmaceuticals or using some other biomedical approach, what can we do to increase and activate sirtuins? Remember Dr. Kellogg's insistence on eating fresh food but not too much of it, exercising, and looking after your gut health? If you do all the right things, like eating right and exercising, you can repair your DNA. If you do bad things, like smoking, you are negatively altering your DNA.

The Guardians of the Genome Are the Sirtuins

Remember the elevator in the luxury hotel that is used only in emergencies when all the restaurants are closed? That is the sirtuins pathway. That pathway makes sure that the hotel's guests are taken care of when no food is around. That elevator may even get rid of the bad guests at the hotel that are yelling a lot, playing loud music, and annoying the other guests. The sirtuins pathway does the same—it can get rid of the old disruptive cells that are secreting inflammatory toxins. These old cells that are piling up as we age and are disrupting the young cells with inflammatory mediators like interleukin-6.

Sirtuins have had a long and fascinating history as part of our bodies throughout evolution. In prehistoric times, before Whole Foods, Trader Joe's, and other supermarkets provided us with an endless variety of readily available food and tasty snacks, food was scarce. Early humans didn't have it so easy. They had to endure starvation for extended periods of time. They needed a huge reserve of energy to effectively hunt big animals like mammoths and buffaloes. Protein sources were scarce. They had to survive harsh environments like extreme heat and cold.

It's important to note that any extreme condition stresses the body. This is when sirtuins get their moment to shine. At the most basic level, sirtuins are survival triggers. Their job has always been to recognize when we are experiencing physical stress and then kick up gene activity to work at their most effective levels to keep us alive. Adversity was key for longevity.

For example, sirtuins get activated with extreme temperatures. Extreme cold for prolonged periods of time will result in frostbite. You can lose your extremities and die from an infection or sepsis. If, however, you are in extreme cold for a shorter period, you will still be incredibly uncomfortable, but your sirtuins will boost your immune system to fight off whatever could kill your cells. Again, it is like that emergency elevator I talked about. This emergency elevator is bringing the hotel's guests blankets to endure the cold and stay warm when the heater is out and there are extreme cold temperatures in the building. Or when the air conditioner is out and the temperature is too hot, the emergency elevator will bring the hotel's guests buckets of ice and fans to cool them down. Sirtuins do the same. Sirtuins always want to make sure your cells are okay in extreme situations such as hunger, cold, or extreme heat.

Thanks to all the research done on sirtuins, we are now learning how and when to trigger these amazing proteins. We know what triggers all types of sirtuins, which are primarily responsible for DNA repair, creation of energy, and how and when triggers should be activated or shut off.

We are also learning what keeps those incredible sirtuins from getting triggered, diminishing our lifespans and health. We are learning what interferes with sirtuins doing their jobs and leads to chronic disease. Often, it is the constant attacks on our genes by things like UV rays, smoking, excess food, comfortable temperatures, and the introduction of toxins into our bodies.

Sirtuins Are the Cells' CEO

Sirtuins improve cell health and keep things in balance. Think of your cells as a company. For your company to run efficiently, every employee has a different job. There are assistant managers, senior managers, payroll staff, and a CEO. As priorities in the company change, the CEO directs the employees to work differently or more effectively. The same goes for your cells. Sirtuins are your cells' CEO. Sirtuins manage your cells. They tell the cells what to do. They control your life. We can take advantage of this knowledge and find ways to be healthier and to live longer.

To Activate Sirtuins and Have Healthy Cells

- Become more active.
- Get exposed to small bouts of cold or heat.
- Try intermittent fasting.
- Exercise often.
- Avoid chemicals in food and environment.
- Eat food rich in polyphenols (berries, tea, cocoa, nuts, beans, spices, and olive oil).

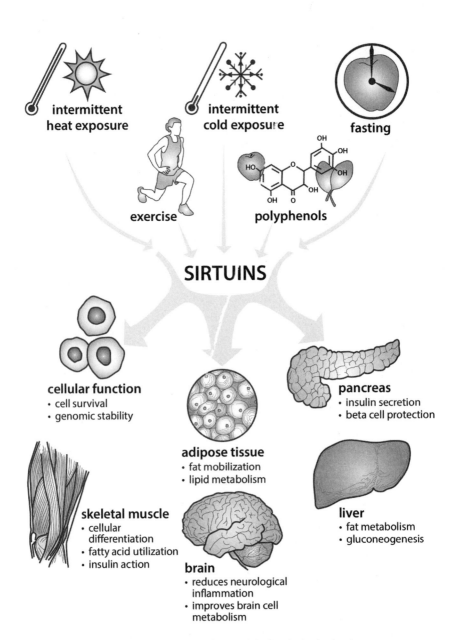

Factors that affect sirtuins and their role in the body.

Just like a good CEO can make a great company, or a director can make a great movie, sirtuins do the same. They affect your longevity when you activate them. Make sure sirtuins are always on your side as you embark on this new ageless journey.

Remember . . .

- *Epigenetics* is the science of how DNA can be altered by diet, life-style choices, and medications.

- *Epigenomes* are a group of chemicals and proteins that attach themselves to DNA, mark it, and leave a record of an activity so that it can be turned on and off in the future.

- Sirtuins are the proteins that keep your cells healthy. To keep sirtuins healthy avoid UV rays, smoking, and unhealthy foods.

- *Sirtuins are also activated by excess heat and cold.*

PART II

Getting Ready to Start *The Ageless Revolution*

CHAPTER 6

Banish Bad Habits

Bad habits are like chains that are too light
until they are too heavy to carry.
—**Warren Buffet**

In 1994, I started my residency training. I was fit and in shape. During residency, medical residents spend two to three nights a week in the hospital working thirty-six-hour shifts or being on call. Sleep deprivation, lack of exercise, and a poor diet took a toll on my health. Within a year, my weight ballooned to 215 pounds from 175 pounds. In no time, I was overweight, short of breath with minimal efforts, and had absolutely no energy whatsoever. I had a "daddy body" at the age of thirty! In 1995, it was a fall day that I will never forget. I was working in the hospital's clinic when one of my patients who saw me a year earlier said to me, "What happened to you, Doc? You used to be so fit!"

Knowing that he was right (unfortunately!), I checked in with a local doctor. My blood tests showed that I now had high cholesterol, insulin resistance, and high sugar. I was prediabetic. Or, in medical terms, I had the metabolic syndrome that 25 percent of Americans have. The doctor advised me to eat less and exercise, but I was exhausted from the insane work schedule and had no time for exercise. Working eighty to ninety hours a week and studying for my board exams left little time to no time to get fit. I must say this was my wake-up call. With three years left on my residency, I knew I had to make some positive changes. First, I stopped treating myself to that cheeseburger and fries that I thought I was entitled to after the thirty-six-hour shifts. It was time to eat right and have more salads. I also stopped munching on those cookies and donuts that the secretaries and nurses always had around. Next, instead of taking the elevator, I started taking the stairs. I trained at Jewish hospital in New York, where they had Shabbat elevators, which stop on every floor on Fridays and Saturdays. So instead of waiting for the elevator for ten minutes each time to take me to my desired floor, whether it was Shabbat or not, I took the stairs all the time. This was my aerobic exercise. I also bought some dumbbells and used them frequently at home. Voilà, I overcame my work challenges. I lost thirty-five pounds in a few months. When I repeated my blood tests, everything normalized. The metabolic syndrome vanished. My health couldn't wait, so I made it a priority. You can do the same, as the best time to take care of yourself is always *right now*! Conquer epigenetic alteration by activating your sirtuins and banishing bad habits. It is time to invigorate your cells.

Removing Obstacles to Better Health

The moral of my story is that on the road to health, the biggest obstacles are the ones you place in your own way, not the ten hallmarks of aging. You can be your own worst enemy. You know the excuses. I'm too busy to work out. I am too tired to work out. Eating healthy is too expensive. I do not know where to begin. I will start on Monday. I am too young to care. Often, these types of mental obstacles can be harder to conquer than the ten hallmarks of aging. No person can remove those mental obstacles for you; only you can. Take responsibility for your own choices. Eliminate "I can't" from your vocabulary.

It may feel like the people in your life are sabotaging your health efforts too. You start a new diet, but your coworker shows up with donuts, brownies, or a birthday cake. You eat them! You are disciplined all week, but a relative calls to invite you to a birthday party, ice cream, or happy hour. You go! You'll need support during this time of your life, so start by telling people you love that you are making changes, so you'll be healthier and live longer. There is absolutely nothing wrong about being known as a health nut. It is your life.

Kick Bad Habits and Change Your Genetic Destiny

It is time to change your genetic destiny. You can do it by getting rid of your bad and unhealthy habits now—the habits that alter your genome or DNA. Having unhealthy habits does not make you bad, lazy, or weak; it makes you human. The two main factors that contribute to forming habits, specifically bad ones, are stress and boredom.

Stress Is a Silent Killer

Stress can come from any part of your life: work, kids, caring for elderly parents, getting an education, or even dating. Often, though, we judge ourselves when we react to stressors. Talk about a vicious cycle! Constant information, stimulation, and entertainment are available to you from a myriad of digital sources, in the palm of your hand, on the table, on the nightstand, in your pocket—just *everywhere*. Boredom can be a problem too. Having downtime can feel scary. You might feel lost or that you are lacking something.

Bad Habits Relieve Stress and Boredom— but at a Cost

Stress and boredom are not pleasant feelings, and it is human nature to do what we can to alleviate any negative feelings we have. To pacify ourselves, we turn to whatever will make us feel good for the moment. Western societies put a premium on feeling good and being happy. The media tells us how we can feel good right now: if we do X, we'll feel Y, much of which isn't good for us. But when you feel down, it's easy to fall into bad habits. Feel sad? Eat some comfort foods or have some of grandma's lasagna that she made just to cheer you up. But if you do this every day, it becomes an eating pattern that can lead to obesity. And obesity is a path to a myriad of illnesses: type 2 diabetes, arthritis, an increased risk for cancer, and a shortened lifespan.

Dealing with a breakup? Go on a bender with friends who want you to have a wild night, forget your heartache, and have a few drinks. Will this one night of binge drinking kill you? No. But if you make it a habit, excess consumption of alcohol can raise your blood pressure and increase your cancer risk.

Staying up late every night to catch up on the latest series on Netflix or one of *The Real Housewives* shows? This alters the production of the hormone melatonin. Melatonin is not only a sleep hormone, but also a major antioxidant that protects the mitochondria, the batteries of your cells. Remember, mitochondria dysfunction is one of the ten hallmarks of aging.

Your boss yells at you. Your reaction: you feel worthless. You need to feel better, so you seek comfort. You might go out and smoke a cigarette, or even a few cigarettes, to perk you up. Now you are altering your DNA, which can lead to cancer. When that self-soothing pattern is repeated often enough, your brain expects it. Do all these actions make you feel better? Yes! But the feeling doesn't last, so you do it again. Often this is how bad habits are born. In no time, you are altering the interpretation of your genome. Like Whitney Houston's analogy that I gave you earlier, you are missing your chance for stardom.

All of this self-soothing repeated behavior can be harmful. For example, as we've seen, overeating to stuff down negative feelings and become numb can lead to obesity, diabetes, other physical infirmities, and death. Gambling can mean you lose money, jeopardize your family's security, and end meaningful relationships. This actually leads to more stress or poor sleep. Smoking can open the door to lung cancer and other respiratory problems.

We all engage in unhealthy habits that have different degrees of negative effects on our bodies. But if you do not address them now, all the guidance in this book will not help you. You can blow into a balloon all you like, but if there is a pinprick in it, it simply won't inflate. Bad habits are that pinprick, and they can sabotage your health and longevity.

Getting Rid of Bad Habits

You need your sirtuins to be fired up, to be turned on. One of the best ways to do this is by kicking bad habits. But it won't happen overnight. Adopting good habits takes time. There's no quick tap of a magic wand to make it happen just like that. But committing to retraining your mind and body is essential to success in *The Ageless Revolution.*

Start Small Changes to Create a Huge Impact

I don't expect you to kick all your bad habits all at once as you start on *The Ageless Revolution* but take baby steps. If you set your expectations of yourself too high, you will feel bad and sabotage yourself. Remember, you are reversing years, if not decades, of learned unhealthy behavior. Be patient and kind to yourself. Give your body and your brain the time they need to detox, reset, and restore. Eventually, your health and metabolism will respond positively to every change you make. Ridding yourself of these bad habits gives you the best chance of success, health, and longevity with *The Ageless Revolution.*

Smoking

With marijuana being legalized across the country in state after state, more people are smoking (or just now admitting to) pot on a regular basis. Stop! Smoking is the most damaging thing you can do to age fast. Smoking kills four hundred thousand Americans every year. It harms your cells, organs, and genes. It damages your DNA and your lungs too. Smoking ages you by decades, not just years. Outside of industrial carcinogens (such as asbestos or chemicals found in the pesticides used in commercial farming), nothing wreaks havoc on your health like the chemicals in cigarettes because they alter your DNA.

Smoking damages your cell walls with free radicals, which leads to impaired cellular communications. You can take control of these two hallmarks of aging in a big way by kicking the habit. While you can't control toxic substances in your environment, you can control what you put in your body. So do whatever you have to do to quit. It will extend your life expectancy and reduce your risk of developing a chronic illness. Heart disease, COPD, and cancer are all linked to smoking. Quitting will immediately improve your heart and respiratory health. Talk to your doctor about the variety of medications that are available to help you quit. But is vaping okay? In a single word, no. Vaping may be less damaging to your health than smoking, but it is still not good for you. The key ingredient in vape cartridges is nicotine, which makes vaping just as addictive and damaging as smoking. Some smokers say they were able to get off cocaine more easily than they were able to get off nicotine. Vaping tastes good and pumps you up, but it is doing cellular damage you want to avoid. Keep your lungs and respiratory system as clean and healthy as possible.

Sugar

Stop eating refined sugar. Period. Refined sugar is devoid of nutrients, is inexpensive, and can be found in baked goods like cupcakes, donuts, cereal, and all types of processed foods. It's also found in so-called healthy foods such as sweetened yogurt—which has loads of added sugar. High-fructose corn syrup, a cheap form of sugar, is often a main ingredient in pancake syrups, puddings, canned fruits, and more.

The Problem with Sugar

Sugar raises insulin, which is linked to weight gain and inflammation. Both high insulin and insulin resistance are linked to a shortened lifespan. Research has also shown that being overweight or obese increases the risk of several types of cancers, including breast, colorectal, pancreatic, and ovarian cancer. The damage does not stop here. Too much sugar raises your cholesterol and damages your arteries. Think if you ever dropped soda or honey on the floor, it is very hard to clean. It is very sticky and messy. Sugar does the same inside the body. It sticks to cholesterol and hardens your arteries. It can lead to early Alzheimer's disease. The increase of glucose in your body from eating refined sugar can lead to obesity, type 2 diabetes, liver disease, heart disease, and stroke. Eating sugar also tricks your body into turning off its appetite-control system, and you gain weight as insulin is secreted in higher amounts. Insulin is a hormone that stores fat.

Sugar also shortens your telomeres. It stunts your stem cells and confuses them. They do not know what to do, so no more regeneration. In other words, your stem cells can't come to the rescue when there is cellular damage. Remember Plastic Man whom I talked about earlier, who can morph into anything you want him to be? With sugar, Plastic Man is paralyzed; he does not know what to do. As doctors, we all have seen how wounds in diabetics don't heal so fast. And here comes the big problem that can shorten lives: excess sugar also stimulates the wrong stem cells, and they can become cancerous. In other words, sugar promotes cancer. Sugar also negatively affects both the IGF-1 and AMPK pathways of nutrient sensing. This leads to their dysfunctions. When these pathways are malfunctioning, cellular damage follows.

Remember the elevators in the hotel I talked about earlier? If those elevators get overused by delivering too much sugar and cookies all the time to the hotel's guests, they will break down. The same goes for those pathways: They get overloaded and get impaired when they are overused with sugar. In turn, the cells suffer.

Sugar also ages your skin more quickly. It damages the collagen in your body as it sticks to the tissues. Collagen encourages new cell growth and turnover. Eat too much sugar, and it promotes wrinkles and damages you from the inside out. Topical creams and serums to increase skin firmness don't stand a chance. So you'll need to tame your sweet tooth for the sake of longevity. Sugar should be an occasional treat; it is not food. Sugar is shunned in all of the five Blue Zones.

The Problem with Soda

Liquid calories are simply not as satisfying as calories we get from solid foods. That is why it is easy for some of us to drink soda after soda all day.

It's not like eating delicious solid food like berries or other fruit. You keep drinking soda and other calorie-laden drinks because your brain is not registering your intake. And you add more calories to your regular diet by guzzling tons of sugary drinks. Fructose found in soda in the form of high-fructose corn syrup is even worse than sugar. Diet sodas are not any better with all the artificial sweeteners.

A Patient's Story

Chris is one of my patients who came to see me for frequent urination. After running some blood tests, Chris was found to be diabetic. Chris weighed 250 pounds and was five feet eight inches tall. He had a body mass index (BMI) of thirty-four (twenty is the normal BMI for men), elevated triglycerides level, and very low levels of high-density lipoprotein cholesterol (C-HDL), all risks for heart disease.

The problem? Chris consumed a massive amount of sugar, without even realizing it! Each morning, Chris had cereal with fat-free milk and orange juice. A usual lunch was a lean ham or chicken sandwich on white bread with fat-free mayo, and baked potato chips. Chris snacked on fat-free yogurts and pretzels. He had pasta for dinner most nights.

Chris thought he was following a healthy low-fat diet as he tried to lose weight. The problem is that he ate practically nothing *but* sugar, which was causing all his health problems. I had Chris change his diet and cut down massively on his sugar intake. Chris started to eat eggs for breakfast, salads for lunch. I made him snack on nuts. Within one year, he was down to a healthy weight, his diabetes resolved with no meds.

Fast Carbs and Processed Foods

Even if you avoid sugar, say you like to eat refined carbohydrates, like a plain bagel for breakfast or pizza or have white rice with dinner. Bad news: refined carbohydrates such as white bread and white rice aren't much better than sugar. In your gut, refined carbs break down into sugar quickly and spike the hormone insulin. In no time, you are hungry again. Too much sugar speeds up cellular aging. It leads to overworking the nutrient pathways. Refined carbs are found in processed and packaged foods. This includes the processes of canning, cooking, freezing, dehydrating, or milling that removes the good fiber from grains. Their nutritional value has been compromised. Not to mention all the added salt, sugar, unhealthy fats, and chemical preservatives.

Chemicals alter your genome, or DNA, and chromosomal instability is one of the ten hallmarks of aging. Chemicals also impair cellular communications, another hallmark of aging. Processed foods negatively affect your nutrition, insulin level, and your longevity. Processed carbohydrates work against your metabolism.

The Danger of Fast Carbs

David Kessler, the former commissioner for the Food and Drug Administration (FDA), coined the expression "fast carbs" to name processed food products that have destroyed the structural integrity of the ingredients. These include white breads, cakes, cookies, crackers, and anything made of white flour. Milled white flour removes the part of the grain that has healthy fiber and nutrients. This is then used in baked goods, which, when eaten quickly, unleash glucose into your bloodstream. Even flour labeled "enriched" is bad. It is just white flour that has been stripped of fiber and any natural nutrients.

Fiber is important because it slows digestion and delivers nutrients on the way. It helps the gut flora, which is important for longevity. Gut health keeps your mitochondria, or the battery of your cells, healthy. Good gut bacteria helps prevent colon cancer.

Why We Need Good Fiber

Gut health is one of the ten hallmarks of aging. Fiber is like a time-release capsule, making sure our systems can absorb nutrients without flooding the blood with sugar. Overprocessing grains and plants removes their natural fibrous structures, turning them into no more than nutrient-poor globs of paste that blast sugar to overwhelm your endocrine system. The destroyed fiber can no longer act like a scrub brush in your intestines. Slower digestion means you would eat less. With refined carbs, you are hungry in no time. It is like eating pure sugar. Think of how you feel when you eat ice cream. Do you want to stop after one scoop? Of course not. It is addicting with the rapid sugar release in the blood. In addition, processed white flour cannot stimulate the digestive tract to keep it clean and healthy. It leads to having bad bacteria in your gut. Gut health is one of the ten hallmarks of aging, and its dysfunction leads to brain issues such as ADHD, autism, and Alzheimer's disease.

Why We Eat Things That Aren't Good for Us

The food industry has made white flour products irresistible by adding tons of sugar, salt, or both. Food scientists know that sugar and salt activate the addictive parts of our brains. Adding sugar and salt-laden chemical flavorings to cardboard-like food creates a sizable population of junk-food addicts. That is why, when we get our hands on a bag of cookies or potato chips, we cannot eat just one. Our brain lights up in all the reward centers, and we want more. Before we know it, we have gobbled down an entire bag of cookies or chips and feel sick and guilty.

Cut junk food from your diet to give your body a fighting chance for health and a longer life. You will feel better about yourself and your food choices. The best way to avoid fast carbs is to keep sugar, processed foods, and junk food away from your house and replace it with healthy alternatives, which you'll learn about here. Get more creative with your salads by adding berries, nuts, and goat cheese. My philosophy on food, health, and longevity is to get rid of unhealthy food and move into a lifestyle defined by using fresh foods as your best fuel.

Sugar, Insulin, and Insulin Resistance

Eating too much sugar can lead to metabolic syndrome, which is the first step for modern diseases that shorten life: heart disease, type 2 diabetes, cancer, and neurodegenerative diseases such as Alzheimer's disease. Think of water flowing in a river. When it rains, the water begins to rise so high that the river overflows. It's the same with sugar. When you eat small amounts of sugar for an occasional treat, it is used for energy, and no problem happens. But when you eat too much sugar, it burdens the organs, and chronic diseases follow.

With so much sugar in the blood, the pancreas has to secrete more insulin. The pancreas gets overwhelmed. In no time, the cells also become insulin resistant, meaning they don't respond to the hormone insulin to let the sugar in. Both insulin and sugar remain high in the blood, which can lead to atherosclerosis and cancer.

Insulin resistance can lead to type 2 diabetes. Diabetes now is the seventh cause of death in the United States. Patients with diabetes have a much greater risk for cardiovascular disease, cancer, and Alzheimer's disease.

Excess sugar is also stored as collagen in the liver and muscles. Collagen is sugar-connected molecules. When your muscles are already full of collagen, this extra sugar is stored as—you guessed it—fat.

Fructose and the Metabolic Syndrome

It is not just sugar that is a problem and making us sick, fructose does too. Fructose in particular is a powerful driver of metabolic syndrome. Fructose is a natural sugar that is present in fruits. But as we evolved, unlike other mammals, we lost an enzyme that breaks down fructose.

Yes, you can eat an orange, and you will be okay because that orange also has fiber, water, and some fructose. But our bodies were not designed to drink quarts of orange juice or soda with massive amounts of high fructose corn syrup. Fructose in the body creates uric acid. High uric acid is related to the metabolic syndrome, high blood pressure, gout, diabetes, and fatty liver. Stay away from fruit juices and soda.

Learn to Respect Your Body

As you learn more about how your body functions, you are going to respect it more and want to keep it in its best working order. You will stay away from sugar, chemicals, artificial flavorings, preservatives—all the ingredients that pollute processed foods and mess up your metabolism, hormones, and cellular communications.

Excess Sun Exposure

Of course, it goes without saying that limiting the time spent under the sun is key to having younger-looking skin. The UV rays of the sun damage your skin and make it look decades older. A little sun is good for us to make some vitamin D. But spending too much time in the sun causes you to have wrinkles, sunspots, and an increased risk of developing skin cancer. The sun damages your DNA, and chromosomal instability is one of the ten hallmarks of aging. I am afraid natural sunscreens do not adequately protect us from the UV rays. Look for sunscreens with bemotrizinol, which is a large molecule that is not absorbed through the skin and protects against UV rays. Unfortunately, bemotrizinol is not FDA approved, so those types of sunscreens are not available in the United States. Look for these products online. Use sunscreen with an SPF of 50. It is quite adequate. Anything more than that does not offer much greater protection and exposes you to chemicals you don't need.

Hard Alcohol

Do you drink a lot? It is time to cut down or stop. In mindful moderation, alcohol is okay (max five to six drinks in a week). In fact, alcohol has a thinning effect on the blood. But in excess, it is terrible for longevity. It is simply liquid sugar. Everything that sugar does to wreak havoc on your body also happens when you ingest alcohol. Alcohol also has more consequences.

The Seven Big Dangers of Alcohol

1. **It prevents your body from doing all its jobs.** Your body is smart enough to want to get rid of alcohol as fast as possible. Alcohol has no

nutritional benefit, and there is no way for your body to store it, as it does with good stuff like protein and carbohydrates. Alcohol is the first thing your body metabolizes, and as your liver detoxes your body to remove alcohol from your blood, you overwork that organ. That is why cirrhosis of the liver is a common disease among alcoholics.

2. **Alcohol can grow bad bacteria in your gut.** That unhealthy bacteria overtakes the good bacteria that produce chemicals that protect the mitochondria. Mitochondrial dysfunction is one of the ten hallmarks of aging. Gut health is also one of the ten hallmarks of aging.

3. **Alcohol leads to heart disease.** Excessive alcohol leads to high blood pressure, which damages the heart, which can lead to heart failure and stroke. Alcohol can directly damage the heart muscle, which in medical terms is called cardiomyopathy.

4. **Alcohol can lead to pancreatitis.** Pancreatic juices have enzymes that break down food. The pancreas also creates hormones that help your metabolism. Excess alcohol leads to pancreatitis, a disease that stops all those important things from happening and eventually leads to early death.

5. **Alcohol can lead to cancer.** The most common cancers caused by excessive alcohol drinking are liver cancer, pancreatic cancer, and breast cancer. Enough said.

6. **Alcohol can damage your immune system.** Chronic drinkers are more susceptible to cold, flu, pneumonia, and other infections.

7. **Alcohol leads to a depletion of stem cells.** Excess alcohol leads to an acceleration or depletion of your stem cells.

Types of Alcoholic Beverages to Drink on *The Ageless Revolution*

Alcohol has a thinning effect on the blood. But not all alcohol is good for us or is the same for longevity. Beer, for example, has an excess of purine, a chemical compound that raises uric acid. High uric acid is linked to a shortened lifespan by three to four years. High uric acid also results from food high in purines, such as certain cheese, meats, and anchovies.

Beer also makes you gain weight because of excess maltose, a sugar that raises insulin and is a fat-storing hormone. High insulin and insulin resistance are linked to a shortened lifespan. If you like to drink beer, at least go for the low-carb variety. Whiskey in moderation lowers uric acid levels. I bet you did not expect a doctor to tell you that a glass of Jack Daniel's is better for your health than a beer. But the best alcoholic drink is red wine. Red wine, in moderation, can have positive effects on health. Plants get stronger when they face adversity, they have more nutrients, and their benefits pass on to us. The skin of the grape is rich in a compound called resveratrol, an antioxidant that can help protect the lining of blood vessels in your heart, reduce low-density lipoprotein cholesterol (LDL, the "bad" cholesterol), and prevent blood clots. It also boosts your heart health. Resveratrol turns on and affects sirtuins. Remember sirtuins are your cells' CEO. They dictate the health of your cells.

Resveratrol has also been found to manipulate longevity genes. In his lab at Harvard University, Dr. David Sinclair, who has been studying the effects of this supplement on health and longevity, gave resveratrol to mice who had been fed a high-calorie diet. Amazingly, those mice did not develop all the diseases associated with that kind of diet. Instead, they had reduced fat cells, more energy and strength, improved coordination and mobility, and lived longer than mice in a control group.

In humans, resveratrol supplementation has been very controversial. Resveratrol works on sirtuin 1 and mimics caloric restriction. But the initial results on mice and worms have not been replicated in many other animal studies. Some scientists argue that resveratrol is not easily absorbed when taken with water and it should only be consumed with some fats like olive oil or full-fat yogurt to see the full benefits. No one knows.

But it appears red wine appears to play a role with longevity and even affects skin health. A particular red wine made with muscadine grapes can give you great-looking skin with more elasticity and water retention. If you think you have a problem with alcohol, talk to your doctor about a variety of medications, treatments, and methods that can help you move beyond your addiction.

Although it is tempting to give into bad habits, making healthy choices is the smart thing to do. Bad habits rarely exist in the five Blue Zones. So it is time to copy their lifestyles and healthy habits. It can make a world of difference. You can choose health and longevity. I end this chapter by borrowing a quote from Viktor Frankl, an Austrian psychiatrist, founder of existential analysis, and a survivor of the Nazi concentration camps, who said, "Forces beyond your control can take away everything you possess except one thing, your freedom to choose how you will respond to the situation."

Remember . . .

- Alter your DNA in a positive way by eliminating or at least decreasing consumption of sugar and fast carbs—all processed foods—and excess alcohol.

- Stop smoking. You will live longer.

- Avoid sugar in all forms.

- Limit the time spent under the sun. Always use sunscreen.

- Avoid indulging in those "I want to feel better now" moments and keep your eyes on the bigger goal of good health and longevity.

CHAPTER 7

The Ageless Revolution Makeover

You can't help getting older, but you don't have to get old.
—**George Burns**

Epigenetic alteration affects your lifespan. Thirty percent of how you age depends on genetics. This means the rest is up to you. Think of Singapore, the manufactured sixth Blue Zone. You can change your genetic destiny. You, alone, control your future.

As you've seen, cutting out junk food and sugar, quitting smoking, and limiting alcohol are all ways to eliminate roadblocks to health and longevity. Your body is an extraordinarily complex machine. More complex than a Ferrari. Hell, it is more complex than a Boeing 787 Dreamliner. In this chapter, we'll tackle a few more problems and unhealthy habits in *The Ageless Revolution* that can negatively affect our cell walls, DNA, and mitochondria and impact health and longevity.

Stress

A common denominator in all five of the Blue Zones is a stress-free life. Stress affects cortisol, which affects insulin, and eventually your metabolism.

A stress-free life is impossible, but you can get a handle on stress with the right measures.

What Is Stress?

"Stress is a normal human reaction that happens to everyone. In fact, the human body is designed to experience stress and react to it.

When you experience changes or challenges (stressors), your body produces physical and mental responses. That is stress. Stress responses help your body to adjust to new situations. Stress can be positive, keeping us alert, motivated, and ready to avoid danger. Stress can give a boost of cortisol to run and avoid getting hit by a car. Or if you have an important test coming up, a stress response might help your body work harder and stay awake longer. But stress becomes a problem when stressors continue without relief or periods of relaxation. When your body is stressed, its autonomic nervous system kicks in. The autonomic system controls your heart rate, breathing, vision, and more. Its built-in stress response, the fight-or-flight response, helps the body face stressful situations. When a person has long-term [chronic] stress, continued activation of the stress response causes wear and tear on the body. Physical, emotional, and behavioral symptoms develop." —*The Cleveland Clinic*

That fight-or-flight feeling comes from an increase of adrenaline and can save you from real and impending danger. It can also put so much strain on your body that you may wind up with chest pain, headaches, high blood pressure, digestive problems, depression, and even a weakened immune system.

Any form of stress—whether it is worry, nervousness, anxiety, or obsessive thinking—triggers your body into "high alert" mode by flooding it with cortisol, a hormone. Too much, too often, and you can become permanently locked in a state of fight-or-flight physiologically.

Our evolution has programmed us to either run or fight when we feel threatened. This serves us in times of danger, but it can make us feel terrible in the moment and long term. Stress can make you run to the emergency room with chest pain and shortness of breath. Stress depletes your body of stem cells. In other words, long-term stress may shorten your life and can kill you.

The Effect of Stress on the Body

When you are stressed, your body is flooded with adrenaline and cortisol whether you are fighting or fleeing, and eventually, you burn out your metabolism. Keep a gas stove burner on high, and, eventually, the fuel will run out and the flame will die. The same goes for your body. You are no longer running from a saber-toothed tiger or getting into hand-to-hand combat, but your body is tricked into thinking you are and that it needs more fuel to manage that burst of extraordinary exertion.

This creates a double whammy for your metabolism, which simultaneously holds onto the fuel it has stored as fat while asking the body to take in more fuel to be ready for that burst of activity. Cortisol and insulin hormones are interlinked, so chronic stress can give you diabetes. High insulin means inflammation. Several studies have linked stress with shorter telomeres. There is also an increased risk for heart disease, type 2 diabetes, and cancer.

My Own Experience with Stress

In life, we all have our ups and downs. Sometimes, we forget the most important thing in life—our health. After I finished my residency, I tried to watch my weight after I lost the excess pounds, but stress stuck up on me. In 2006, I had been in private practice for a few years, and my hands started shaking nonstop. I was having tremors. Around the same time, my dad passed away, and the tremors got much worse. I thought I had Parkinson's disease in my forties.

I wondered how this could happen to me at such a young age. Did I have the genetics for the disease? I consulted with two neurologists, who told me I didn't have Parkinson's but were also not sure what was really wrong with me. I had no diagnosis.

I was bewildered and, worse, couldn't do procedures on my patients for a few months. I looked for alternative treatments, but nothing worked.

Eventually, I developed insomnia and became severely depressed. I started to have some suicidal thoughts. I found myself crying alone for no reason. Nothing gave me joy, and life was not worth living.

I'd never been depressed before and had no history of it in my family. Normally, I'm a very happy and optimistic person.

I wrote myself a script for an antidepressant, but the depressive symptoms did not improve, and the suicidal thoughts persisted. I did not act on them because I thought of my family and my patients. I could not do any harm or hurt to the people who loved me and needed me.

I should have gone for grief counseling right after my dad passed, but I procrastinated. Believe it or not, doctors, most of the time, are the worst patients. My excuse, I had no time. Eventually, after a few months, I decided to see a therapist, hoping she could help me with my grief and depression. She asked me, "Have you ever thought it could all be related to stress?" "Stress!" I replied, "I am not stressed at all." I laughed, thinking she was joking. The therapist's advice was to meditate, relax, clear my mind, and just do nothing for fifteen minutes every night. I reluctantly but religiously followed her advice.

It turned out that she was 100 percent right. The strange thing is that I didn't even know I was stressed! Long hours, the bureaucracy of the practice of medicine, tons of paperwork, and the passing of my father all took a heavy toll on me.

I eventually realized that it was cumulative stress that led to my hand tremors, insomnia, eventual depression, and suicidal thoughts. High cortisol leads to depression by shutting down serotonin, a chemical neurotransmitter that controls our mood, and melatonin, the sleep hormone. Both cortisol and melatonin must be balanced. So it was no wonder that my stress hormones gave me hand tremors, and my lack of sleep led to my depression. It was all in my head.

My New Routine to Reduce Stress and Change My Life

I began to meditate each night for fifteen minutes. I also worked on my sleep hygiene. I established a bedtime and a wake time and stuck to it. I used to stay up late at night watching TV until 1 AM. I used to be sucked into the media's hype and gimmick, saying who was gonna be next on one of the late shows, whether it was *Jay Leno* or *David Letterman*, and could not be missed. I stayed up. Now, I have become the most important person in my life. It was time to go to bed at 10 PM. In less than two weeks, I felt better. My hand tremors were gone, and so was my depression. I was happy and off the antidepressant meds in no time. But something else happened. I decided to create a science-proven plan to turn my life around and live healthily. I made a new beginning after living a few decades on this earth. I became a new man.

Work and Stress

We are all facing stress in our lives, and how we cope with it can have profound consequences. More than half of Americans report that work is a significant source of stress in their lives. Working to earn enough money to survive and maintain a lifestyle is a source of daily struggle for everyone.

Almost every job also has some sort of stress. Doctors have one of the highest suicide rates of all professions even though they earn a decent income. Through my own struggle I learned to reduce my stress and change my life. You can do that too.

Today, my job doesn't define me. What does is how I can make things better for those I love and positively affect my patients' lives. I had a purpose. People in the Blue Zones have daily rituals that reduce stress, such as prayer, napping, and happy hour. You can follow in their footsteps.

So, get a handle on your stress. Life is so precious. If it is money that is stressing you out, get out of the rat race, cut down on your expensive lifestyle, or get a second job. You don't need every dress or pants in the mall. You don't need every channel on your TV. For daily stress, treat yourself to a professional massage or ask your partner to give you one, and you can reciprocate. Take a hot bath rather than a shower. Learn to meditate every day for at least fifteen minutes. Do whatever you need to do. There are all kinds of health resources available to help you get rid of stress with no extra money needed. Explore apps, YouTube, and the Internet. Or listen to some relaxing music. No excuses! I truly want *The Ageless Revolution* to turn your life around.

Grounding to Handle Stress

Everything is made of energy. Our bodies interact with earth since we showed up on earth. Grounding is touching the earth barefoot to connect with its electrical energy. The idea is that when you touch the ground barefoot, it dissipates electricity and extracts charges that are in you while, at the same time, you receive a charge of energy from free electrons, helping your body synchronize with the natural frequencies of the earth. This practice is rooted in the theory that the electrical charges from the earth can have a positive impact on the body, health, and mood. Initially, I was a skeptic on grounding, but I found a few studies that show its benefits. In our modern times, we wear shoes, and we are isolated from earth. These small studies have reported benefits for inflammation, pain, mood, and much more. Research shows it helps with joint pain and improves mood. Is it a placebo effect? Do people who do grounding feel more connected to nature so they are less stressed? No one knows. Surprisingly, the people who do grounding have longer telomeres. You can do grounding by walking on grass barefoot, walking on a beach, or gardening. Be careful of your surroundings. You can get bit by insects or get poison ivy. But you can do grounding also indoors by using a mat that keeps you connected to earth. It is meditation time. Use a conductive pillow or mat that you can buy online. Do whatever you have to do to get a handle on your stress.

Poor Sleep

I shared with you my personal story to show you how far stress affected me and my sleep. Poor sleep is one of the things that was ignored for too long in the medical profession. Fortunately, for the last two decades, sleep is finally getting the attention it deserves for longevity. During sleep, all our cellular and regulatory systems, including our metabolism, recharge and recalibrate.

The American Academy of Sleep Medicine and the Sleep Research Society recommend adults get at least seven hours of sleep a night. Over one-quarter of adults do not meet this recommendation. About 10 percent of adults suffer from long-lasting insomnia. In order for us to fall asleep, this happens when a hormone called melatonin is secreted. But melatonin is not just a sleep hormone; it is also the most important antioxidant in our body and helps support healthy mitochondria, which produce energy. Melatonin is produced and stored in the pineal gland, which is under the brain, but it is also inside the cells in the mitochondria.

When melatonin levels are depleted, you suffer from insomnia. And *that* is a sign of trouble ahead. Mitochondrial dysfunction is one of the ten hallmarks of aging. Sleep deprivation is related to a variety of illnesses, including weight gain, cardiovascular disease, stroke, and cancer. When your circadian rhythm (the twenty-four-hour internal clock that regulates cycles of alertness and sleepiness) is disrupted because of poor sleep, it ultimately affects your hormones and immune system. Poor sleep triggers a cascade of negative consequences from insulin resistance to cognitive decline.

Many studies show the high cost to the health of night shift workers, who experience higher rates of obesity and higher rates of disease onset, including diabetes, heart disease, and cancer, because their sleep is disrupted. All of this is related to mitochondrial dysfunction.

Quality Sleep and Metabolic Health

Getting adequate rest, in regular, uninterrupted blocks of sleep, is essential to supporting metabolic health. Our metabolism is calibrated to function on an awake/sleep cycle synchronized with the twenty-four-hour day/night cycle. You must keep that circadian rhythm to have a healthy sleep cycle. That is why getting an average of seven to eight hours of sleep is essential to support overall health, body weight, and longevity.

Practice Good Sleep Hygiene

It is important to make your bed a sanctuary. Even minimal light inhibits melatonin secretion. Break the habit of being too attached to all the screens around you. Turn off the television, your cell phone, and your tablet at least one hour before going to bed. The LED blue lights from electronic devices are bad for melatonin secretion. Melatonin is also inhibited by nearby electromagnetic fields that come from cell phones, computers, lamps, electric alarm clocks, and electric blankets. Use ear plugs if your bedroom is noisy. Also establish regular sleep and wake times. Try to go to bed no later than 10 PM, maybe at 11 PM on weekends. Try to get at least seven hours of sleep each night.

In addition to those external factors, give your digestive system time to finish its job. Do not eat too close to bedtime. Usually, eating two or even three hours before sleep is good practice. Exercise during the day, not before you crawl into bed. You want your metabolism to calm down, not rev up. Quality sleep is not only essential; it is one of the most important tools for longevity.

Are You Sleeping Too Much?

If you find yourself sleeping more than eight hours a day, this may be a sign of an underlying health issue, like depression or an underactive thyroid. Trim your sleep time back to eight hours and take note of how that makes you feel. If you are unable to do this, or you find yourself chronically tired, see your doctor as soon as possible. Also avoid taking melatonin supplements if you can. Supplementation of melatonin can suppress your own natural production of that important hormone. Attempt to boost your levels naturally by implementing good sleep hygiene. If you have trouble falling asleep, avoid caffeine at least five hours before bedtime, limit alcohol, and have a hot bath before going to bed.

Inactivity

If you want your sirtuins, the CEOs of your cells, turned on, you need to be active. You've probably heard the expression "sitting is the new smoking," which means being sedentary isn't good for your health. The good news is that there's plenty you can do to become more active. Fitness trackers and apps can help you assess how active you are and make positive changes. Move your body as much as possible. Copy the folks in the Blue Zones.

Even though we're no longer hunter-gatherers, we are still mammals that are designed to be in motion. We're just not built to sit and stare at screens for hours on end, and it's not good for us. When we sit for lengthy periods of time, our muscles atrophy, our circulatory systems become sluggish (often dangerously so—think of people who suffer from blood clots because of sitting for a long time during long flights), and our bodies go into metabolic slow motion to hang onto the energy we are not using. That unused energy becomes fat. So get going! Get up and move! Shake your system awake and wake your metabolic system out of its deep slumber.

Overeating

The real value of caloric restriction research lies in its relationship to longevity. When we overeat, we negatively affect the pathways for nutrient sensing. They get overworked. The AMPK pathway is like the low-fuel light on the dashboard of your car. It senses when there are less nutrients. Once there is no food, it activates. It is also activated by exercise. It tells the cells to conserve energy until the food and nutrients are back. It induces the production of new mitochondria. More importantly, the AMPK pathway inhibits mTOR. All good things for longevity. All these positive things are turned off with overeating.

When food is scarce, the body focuses on survival. It tells you, "Stick around longer, live longer in this world to look after your children." When you overeat, you are telling your body, "No need to stay in this world longer since food is abundant." Evolution truly does not care how long you will live on this earth. It is how your DNA was designed. It's up to you to trick it. Overeating is easy to do, even if we do eat a healthy diet. We live in such a supersize culture with portions that can feed two people or more.

Think about the last time you went out for pasta. Was your plate or bowl overflowing with food? Were you served tons of bread before the main course? Was your salad splashed with lots of dressing? That pasta also comes smothered in olive oil and cheese and is far too good to resist, so we overeat.

Our overeating also comes from a lack of portion control. This happens in sneaky ways, such as when we have two or three pieces of toast instead of one at breakfast, or we order the twelve-ounce filet instead of the six-ounce filet when we go out to dinner. We may not even be that hungry, but for sure we are not gonna waste it. Before the steak, we also ate two slices of white bread and devoured an appetizer. Don't forget the alcoholic drink or two before dinner and the decadent, sugary chocolate dessert topped with ice cream and whipped cream.

Unintentional overeating happens in restaurants, drive-throughs, and when we go to a friend's house for dinner, not to mention in our own homes. Abundant food is mistakenly perceived as a fair value or an act of generosity, when in fact, it is excess calories that usually go to your waistline.

Gluttony is an insult to your health, figure, and longevity. From now on, make it a habit to downsize instead of supersize every time you are eating out. Make it a habit to go home with a doggie bag every single time you eat at a restaurant. Think of it as your delicious lunch or dinner for the next day. You will lose weight and save money. As you assess your eating habits during this journey toward health and longevity, check in with yourself and be honest about how much and how often you eat. Keep your eyes on the goal.

Snacking

Just like overeating, snacking turns off the sirtuins, which is certainly not a good thing. You need the repair systems of your cells activated. Snacking is a subgroup of overeating. Many people believe that eating at regular intervals throughout the day—three meals *plus snacks*—is the best way to keep your metabolism fired up and functioning. I totally disagree. Snacks—healthy ones—are optional, not essential.

In fact, intervals between food and intermittent fasting turn on sirtuins, the proteins that affect your genes and longevity. Frequent eating shuts them down, so avoid eating between your big meals. Eating within an eight-hour period may be your best chance for longevity and survival.

What We Can Learn From Other Cultures Beyond the Blue Zones

In *The Ageless Revolution,* I have shared with you longevity lessons from around the world. So now I will take you to the Middle East. In this region, smoking rates are high, at about 20 percent. Sugar is also consumed in excess, but fasting is practiced for religious reasons during Ramadan, the Islamic month when people eat only from sunset until dawn for one month. In this month, Muslims eat and drink nothing for sixteen hours. This acts as a form of intermittent fasting. Cancer rates in the Middle East are 75 to 80 percent lower than in the Western world. Although people in this part of the world tend to overeat a lot of calories in those eight hours, this type of fasting still reduces cancer risk. On the other hand, frequent and excessive eating increases your cancer risk, especially with certain foods: processed meats, overcooked foods, and fried foods.

Snack the Right Way

So, should you abstain from snacking? Of course not. Snacking can improve energy. Smaller units of healthy snacks can be like mini bombs that explode with healthy protein or slow carbs between meals to keep your energy going and your system functioning. Think raw vegetables, fresh fruit, a handful of nuts, or some fiber-dense legumes.

Unhealthy snacking is the kind of eating that goes on all day long and particularly at night after school or work. You may hit the vending machine for a candy bar, eat the donuts a coworker brought to work, nibble on cookies, or dive into a buttery bowl of popcorn after dinner while you binge-watch the latest trending show or movie on Netflix.

Mindless eating is not related to hunger, it can be to keep boredom at bay or because the food offers you some emotional comfort. Often, snack foods are just empty calories. Think of Doritos, barbecue potato chips, cheese crackers, mini-chocolate bars. These items are not food; they contain fillers and chemicals that will do nothing to prolong your life and everything to cut it short.

A Patient's Story

Stephanie is one of my patients who is in her late fifties. She was married to a man who was neither loving nor affectionate. She told me it was a sexless marriage for twenty years, and she felt unloved. Stephanie was 200 pounds and stood at 5 feet 8 inches. She had elevated blood pressure and high cholesterol. She had a demanding job in New York City and had no time to exercise. While her blood pressure and cholesterol levels were kept in check with medications, she couldn't lose the pounds no matter how hard she tried.

When her weight and sugar had gone up a little higher, I confronted her about her diet. It turned out that Stephanie dealt with her marital issues by overeating. It was her comfort. With her weight up, I had to give her some tough love. I asked her whether she saw herself staying married to the same man and being unhappy for the rest of her life. She answered me quickly with a resounding NO!

About ten months later, Stephanie came back to see me, and I was pleasantly surprised. Stephanie was totally transformed: She had lost fifty pounds. She had a new hairdo and wore a stylish dress, and, beyond her appearance, she was absolutely radiating joy.

I questioned her about what she had done differently. She told me that my question was her wake-up call. She filed for divorce, moved out, and was dating a great guy who was crazy about her. She was ecstatic. When I did her blood workup, everything came back normal. Her sugar and cholesterol were all within normal limits. I stopped all her meds.

Her barrier to health was her mind. My question opened her eyes to take a new direction that gave her a healthier lease on life.

Remember . . .

- Stress, poor sleep, inactivity, overeating, and snacking are road-blocks to longevity. They negatively affect your genome by epigenetic alteration.
- Try to reduce and manage stress. Take a walk, meditate, get a massage.
- Grounding can be a way to manage stress. Do it safely indoors.
- Get quality sleep to recharge and recalibrate your body.
- Move. Being physically active is essential for good health and longevity.
- Be mindful of overeating. Watch how much you put on your plate. Snacking counts as overeating, and most of the time it stems from boredom, not hunger.

CHAPTER 8

Effect of Popular Diets on the Hallmarks of Aging

If it doesn't make sense, it's not true.
—Judge Judy

The New Mantra in the 2020s Should Be a Pro-Aging Diet

The U.S. weight-loss industry reached $90 billion in 2023. It is estimated to grow to $150 billion by 2033. You would think with all this expenditure, we would be healthy as a nation. But we are not! Why? It is simple: Those popular diets don't work. I want to tackle every obstacle standing in your way, so let me ask you about your diet: Which diet are you following now?

Every decade has what is in fashion and what is in vogue—the newest diet that people think is the best thing since electricity. In the 1970s, it was all about very-low-fat diets. There was the Pritikin Diet, which is 70 percent carbs. There was also the Dean Ornish Diet, which is also 70 percent carbs. Cereals, potatoes, and bread are what you should eat. In the 1980s and 1990s, it was all about Atkins or low-carb diets; carbs were down to a minuscule 20 percent net carbs a day. Bacon, sausage, and ham are what you should eat. In the early 2000s, it was all about the South Beach Diet. The carbs were up a little, but the butter changed to soybean oil, and the bacon became Canadian bacon. Leaner processed meats and vegetable oils are what you should eat. Hydrogenated fats made it into the diet's products. In 2010, it was back to the recycled idea of keto diets from 100 years ago. Eat salads with cheese and bacon bits to lose weight. Keto diets continue to be all the rage in many books and magazines. How can all sugar and chemicals be good for you?

In the 2020s, we know more. We should be following a pro anti-aging diet based on the latest science. This means a balanced diet with the right amounts of protein, good carbs, healthy fats, and no chemicals. You need to eat less animal products. This is a diet that is good for your hormones, a diet that is good for your cells and DNA to flourish—most importantly, a diet that is good for the ten hallmarks of aging.

Most popular diets do not make any sense, but we foolishly follow them in the belief we are making healthy choices. We eat excess sugar and chemicals added to low-fat products to make them taste better. We eat processed meats such as bacon with added carcinogens because they're low in carbs. We eat frozen entrées that have been in supermarkets' refrigerators for years thanks to preservatives to cut down on calories. Does any of this make sense to you? Of course not. No wonder "unexplained" weight gain is a problem for many people. Rising obesity rates are caused by more sugar, refined carbohydrates, and chemicals.

The food industry lobbied to change dietary guidelines. The result? Many Americans are now addicted to food with added sugar, salt, and chemicals because it makes food crunchy, salty, or sweet. This leads to excess calories and weight gain. We want to be healthier, so we try the latest diet whether it's low-carb, low-fat, or keto. But on the whole, these are not healthy diets! You've seen that the countries with the longest lifespans follow mostly a plant-based diet with minimal animal products.

My greatest wish is to correct what people think is healthy. That is why I wrote *The Perfect 10 Diet* a few years ago. But correcting dietary guidelines is not the job of a single physician; it is the job of medical institutions and medical organizations. But I took the challenge because many of those guidelines, including the ones from prestigious Ivy League institutions, were endangering my patients' health.

Why Expert Guidelines for What to Eat Are Wrong

Plain and simple, the guidelines for what to eat are wrong because they have been influenced by food lobbyists. Take a look at the Harvard Food Pyramid. In the base, you'll find soybean oil, a manufactured fat, as a foundation of a healthy diet. Wrong. Soybean oil must be eliminated and totally avoided. It should not be part of any diet. So should refined vegetable oils such as corn and cottonseed oils. Walk down supermarket aisles, and you will see shelves stocked with refined vegetable oils, a mix of corn, soy, and cottonseed oils. The labels tell you one thing, but these oils are not good for you. These oils create free radicals when they are heated, so they damage the cell walls. Not a good thing when you are trying to protect your cells. The danger does not stop here.

For example, soybean oil can contain trans fats even with no hydrogenation. Hydrogenation is a manufacturing process that adds a hydrogen atom under pressure to make the oil more stable. Trans fats clog arteries and promote cancer. Think of it this way: Trans fats are like plastics. Would you eat plastics? Of course not, but when you eat French fries from your favorite fast-food restaurant, trans fats incorporate in your cell walls and block the nutrients from entering.

The Problem with Trans Fats

Trans fats like those found in fast-food oils stun your stem cells, which, remember, are like Plastic Man, who can morph into anything you want him to be. With refined vegetable oils, the stem cells get confused. They do not know what to do or how to act on becoming the new cells you need them to be. Not only are they stunted, but there is also no regeneration.

Vegetable oils also damage your DNA. Scientists have even discovered that cooks who inhale the fumes from these heated oils also damage their DNA. Just by stepping into a fast-food restaurant you're already accelerating your aging and damaging your DNA.

What Are Trans Fats and Why It Matters

According to the WHO, 5 billion people are at increased risk of heart disease and early death due to trans fats. Developed by chemists in the early part of the twentieth century, margarine and trans fats quickly rose to prominence as cheaper alternatives to butter and animal fats. Until the 1990s, they were widely promoted as healthy fats by the medical establishment. All this has been debunked. Margarine was invented in France in the 1850s to replace butter. Margarine is made by hydrogenation of refined vegetable oils or adding a hydrogen atom under pressure to vegetable oils.

In addition, free radicals result from the extraction process of refined oils or when they are heated. This can damage cell walls and impair cellular communications—a double whammy. The nutrients cannot go inside the cells with the extra hydrogen from the hydrogenation process embedded in the cell walls, blocking their entrance. Your cells need natural fats such as butter in their walls, not fake fats.

Why do we follow these diets? Erroneous and unhealthy recommendations are everywhere. Look at the Mayo Clinic position on processed foods! "Eat egg beaters, have nonfat milk, and liquid margarine! Liquid margarine is better for your health than solid margarine!" That is jaw-dropping advice to hear from another prestigious institution! Liquid margarine is often made with soybean oil. Eggbeaters have soybean oil, too. Sometimes, it is even hydrogenated! Margarine and fake, ultra-processed food should never be part of your diet. Period. With such unhealthy guidelines and dangerous popular diets, your longevity plan does not stand a chance, and all the guidance in this book will not help. In fact, those dangerous guidelines can harm your health and shorten your life. Stay away from all man-made oils.

Just Say No to Fad Diets

There are four popular diet plans that most people try to follow. All of them are problematic when it comes to health. Here's why:

Low-Fat Diets

The problem with low-fat diets is that they have too much sugar and condemn most fats. Low-fat products with added sugar are considered healthy by the public when they are not. Low-fat diets raise insulin, a fat-storing hormone. It is no wonder that once you eat a processed cereal or a plain bagel for breakfast, you are hungry long before it is lunch time. Low-fat diets are also bad for leptin, a hormone that affects your appetite. They are also bad for cortisol, human growth hormone (or HGH), and the sex hormones. Hormones must be in harmony, or poor health follows. Cells need to communicate, and they communicate with hormones. Think of your hormones like musicians that make beautiful music in an orchestra. All musicians must play the same tune and symphony. But what happens when one or two musicians are out of tune? No beautiful music can be heard. Hormonal imbalance is not a joke. But let us see the effect of low-fat diets on the ten hallmarks of aging.

Low-Fat Diets and Excess Sugar

Sugar is detrimental to the AMPK pathway. When this pathway is overloaded, it gets impaired. Deregulated nutrient sensing is one of the ten hallmarks of aging. In addition, the types of fats that low-fat diets recommend are the bad ones including soybean, corn, and cottonseed oils. Often, butter imitations are recommended in these diets, but research shows the danger of those fake fats.

Unnatural refined vegetable oils will not help you live a longer life. I do not care if the margarine is hydrogenated or not, liquid or solid. Avoid all fake fats. Man-made refined vegetable oils damage your DNA and stun your stem cells. It is time to throw away that "I Can't Believe It's Not Butter." I just explained to you why.

How did low-fat diets even become popular, given all these serious health issues? In the 1970s, George McGovern, a U.S. senator from South Dakota, ran for president against Richard Nixon and lost. McGovern was so popular that even Andy Warhol made his portrait. Along the way, he met Nathan Pritikin, an engineer who promoted a very low-fat/high-carbohydrate diet to fight heart disease, which he believed was caused by saturated fat. Mc-Govern invited Pritikin to testify before the senate committee for heart disease. Together, these two men helped shape the diet industry, leading us to the low-fat dogma where we are now.

In fact, it was McGovern's committee that was behind the birth of the original and disastrous USDA Food Pyramid. This USDA pyramid had grains at its base, to be consumed in abundance with no specification if they are whole grains or refined. Refined carbs break down into sugar quickly in your bloodstream, raise insulin, and make us fat. The base of your diet should never be sugar.

So it's no wonder why, in the Western world, we are so unhealthy and sick. People in many poor countries have a longer lifespan than we do in the rich Western countries. As the medical establishment followed the self-serving food industry and soybean lobbyists, all hospitals and many medical professionals advocate a low-fat approach for healthy living! It is an utter disaster. Those recommendations to eat egg whites, have fat-free yogurt, and cook with soybean oil are beyond dangerous. It is the opposite of what we should follow or do.

Why Low-Fat and Fat-Free Foods Are Bad for You

If you have watched many cooking shows (as I have) or you are just a great cook, you know the golden rule of making something delicious: fat equals flavor.

When food scientists for big corporations create super-low-fat foods, they know they need to make them taste good or they won't sell. Food scientists have two tricks up their sleeves: salt and sugar. But the amount of sugar and salt needed to flavor unhealthy foods is so high that they can result in health problems. For example, overuse of salt can lead to high blood pressure, heart disease, stroke, and calcium deficiency.

Artificial preservatives, artificial flavorings, and potentially harmful chemicals are also used in food processing. You may think that low-fat yogurt is a healthy choice, but take a closer look, and you'll find added sugar, high-fructose corn syrup, and artificial colors. None of this promotes healthy DNA or longevity.

Low fat means that you're not eating enough good fats such as olive oil or butter to help regulate your body's functions and optimize sex hormone production. Low-fat diets overproduce insulin, triggering disease and increasing your hunger levels, which leads to weight gain. High insulin also equals inflammation, a catalyst for aging and disease development.

What's Inflammaging?

With cell damage, inflammation occurs. Inflammation or inflammaging is what happens when the old cells do not die and stick around. This a new hallmark of aging that was added in 2022 when scientists learned that old cells secrete toxic chemicals. However, a diet with a suitable amount of natural fat (butter, avocados, full-fat milk) increases the production of sex hormones in your body that keep you looking younger and keep age-related diseases at bay. Fake food is never the answer.

Yes, Saturated Fats Are Actually Good For You

I am probably one of the few doctors in the world that dare to say saturated fats are good for you since they are condemned by the medical establishment in favor of fake fats. How did we arrive at this medical fraud! The information about saturated fats being bad for you comes from Mazola, Crisco, and Fleishmann's. All these manufacturers produce man-made fats. Ancel Keys, a scientist who came up with the saturated fat theory in the 1950s knew it was nonsense, yet he gave in to the soybean lobby as they attacked his theory to preserve their profits.

"The Seven Countries Study," the largest in the twentieth century that Keys conducted starting in 1958, was a total fraud. The study showed that eating saturated fat is linked to heart disease. The countries that Keys chose were cherry-picked just to prove his faulty theory. He wanted to show the superiority of the Mediterranean diet (Italy and Greece). Keys ignored to pick up the Masai of Kenya. A field survey of 400 Masai men and women indicates no clinical evidence of heart disease or atherosclerosis despite a long continued diet of exclusively milk and meat. What about the French? Another country that keys had not picked was France. The French eat plenty of saturated fats such as butter and have a very low rate of heart disease as well. The list just goes on; Switzerland was skipped.

Saturated fats are eaten in abundance by the Swiss too. Switzerland, famous for its cheese fondue dish (melted cheese), has one of the highest life expectancy rates in the world at 84.25 years. In fact, Switzerland is ranked at number four in longevity right after Monaco, Hong Kong, Macao, and Japan. I did a Google search for longevity in 1960, and to my surprise Greece was at number 29 at the time, and Italy was at the number 33 spot! Iceland was at number one. What did people do before Google? Why was there no fact-checking done by doctors or medical journals in the 1960s? Books did exist! Nevertheless, Keys made it to the cover of *Time* magazine in 1961, solidifying his place in history and mistruths.

Exposing the Lie About Dietary Cholesterol and Heart Disease

No relationship exists between dietary cholesterol and heart disease either. Even in a 1997 interview Keys admitted that "there is no connection whatsoever between cholesterol in food and cholesterol in blood." The medical establishment has finally debunked this notion after sixty years! But the damage was enormous.

Sixty years of flawed research led people to fear natural food. But many people aren't aware of these facts. They don't know that eating shrimp is better than eating a dish of grilled lean meat (heterocyclic amines are formed with grilling). Or that whole milk is healthier than low-fat or skim milk because the vitamins found in whole milk are lost during the elimination of fats and added back again.

Consuming fat-free dairy was even linked to infertility in women in a Harvard study. Eggs are better for your health than egg whites. This is because the fatty yolk of eggs is where you find the highest concentrations of fat-soluble vitamins like D, E, and beta-carotene. A low-fat diet can lead to a deficiency in vitamins A and K. Vitamin A increases levels of retinoic acid, which induces stem cells. One of the ten hallmarks of aging is depletion of stem cells. Vitamin K also protects our hearts.

Natural Fat Is Good

When I say, "Fat is good," I mean natural fats like olive oil, nuts, avocados, and butter. Natural fats when eaten in moderation promote satiety and lead to weight loss. Whether you are eating a fat-free yogurt or a fat-free ice cream, the excess sugar and chemicals added to fat-free products to make them tasty creates a sure path to disease.

High-Protein/Low-Carb Diets

When low-fat diets failed, people often went to another extreme: low-carb diets and loaded up on protein. These diets balanced insulin and helped people lose weight. First, what exactly is protein? The word *protein* comes from the Greek word *proteus*, meaning "of first importance." That is precisely what it is. Protein is the basic building block of all tissues and organs and is involved in all chemical reactions in the body. Protein is also needed to relay messages between cells and transport nutrients.

Fish, fowl, eggs, and meat are high in protein. Animal protein is essential to optimize hormone production, but the trick is to eat protein just in the right amounts. I recommend making it only 10 to 15 percent of your diet, depending on your activity level—not 50 percent like low-carb diets! I really don't see 5 percent of protein as eaten in the Blue zones to be adequate because as we age, we lose muscle mass. We need to preserve muscle mass.

A diet *moderate in protein* is key to longevity, *not a diet higher in protein.* Excess protein stimulates the mTOR pathway, which we should slow down as we age. I talked earlier about the elevator in the hotel that transports food from the steak house or restaurant. If this elevator is overused to bring steak and pork chops to the guests nonstop, it will break down. The same happens in your cells: overuse of that pathway leads to cellular deterioration. Following a diet with over 50 percent of the calories coming from protein is far from *a balanced approach.*

You may say, I should become a vegetarian to live longer. No, you will never find a centenarian who is a vegetarian. Animal products contain vitamin B12, which lowers homocysteine, a protein that makes cholesterol sticky. Vegetarians usually have low levels of vitamin B12. Again, balance is the key.

The History of the Low-Carb Diets

The low-carb concept is not new at all; in fact, it has been around for over 200 years. An obese Englishman named William Banting, an undertaker to royal families and elite society, detailed in his book *Letter on Corpulence* how to lose weight by eating an abundance of meat protein and avoiding, even eliminating, starch and sugar. At five feet, five inches tall, Banting initially weighed 202 pounds, but after a year on a low-carb diet, with most of that time voluntarily in a hospital, his weight dropped to 156 pounds. No one knew at the time how those types of diets worked since the hormone insulin had not yet been discovered. We now know that it worked because it lowered insulin, the fat-storing hormone. When you eat eggs and bacon versus eating a bagel with jam your blood sugar levels remain more stable throughout the day, so you eat less.

The late Dr. Robert Atkins was the first in modern times to take note of this ancient low-carb concept and made it popular. Dr. Atkins developed a plan for counting net carbs even from vegetables and fruits. This allowed people to go into ketosis, or to use both fat and protein as a main source for energy.

As a result, high-protein/low-carb diets took off in the 1980s. A sort of renaissance to this 200-year-old approach. I think of the early followers of high-protein/low-carb diets as the earliest biohackers. They succeeded in weight loss and promoted the low-carb lifestyle to the public. A whole industry was built around low-carb products, which contain chemicals like nitrites and other fake ingredients such as soy protein isolate and artificial sweeteners. Dr. Atkins's books were so popular that a plethora of similar low-carb diet books followed over the years. All those copycat low-carb books share the same concept although they may adjust the amount of carbs or fats to eat up or down. Give the book a glamorous location or a catchy sexy title, and you have got the next *New York Times* bestseller.

When you don't eat carbs, you use fat and protein as your main source of energy. Again, you use ketone bodies, which are by-products of fat metabolism. Here is the truth: in reality, most low-carb diet followers never really reach a state of ketosis. If they do reach a state of ketosis, it is for a brief period. The result is just deprivation of delicious carbs. Low-carb followers end up gaining more weight once the carbs are reintroduced.

In 2010, I published my first book, *The Perfect 10 Diet*. It is a balanced diet with no chemicals. The diet was a stark difference from all the popular diets on the market, which tend to be *on* the extremes. In *The Perfect 10 Diet*, I compared low-carb diets to the *Titanic*. The greatness is fake. I still stand by this comparison. The *Titanic* sank on April 15, 1912, four days into her maiden voyage. The ship received six warnings on April 14 that an iceberg was right ahead, but all warnings went ignored. When the iceberg was sighted, she was unable to turn quickly enough. It was too late, resulting in her sinking and the death of 1,500 people. This is my second book, and it is my second warning to the public about high-protein/low-carb diets. I don't see one iceberg, I see several. Get off *now*.

The Dangers of Artificial Sweeteners

The artificial sweeteners in low-carb products like Aspartame or Equal have been linked to cancer. Sucralose or Splenda has been linked to damaged DNA. Erythritol or sugar alcohol has been linked to heart attacks. You might say, "But you have to eat a lot of that, Doc, to suffer from those diseases." True, but the effect is cumulative over a lifetime. How many diet sodas do you drink in one week? How much bacon do you eat in one week when all you are eating is protein? You see my point.

Low-Carb Diets and Gastrointestinal Symptoms

If you follow one of the high-protein/low-carb diets, you will lose weight because you will cut sugar, refined carbs, and balance your insulin. You will eat less because you will be satisfied with less food.

But there are plenty of negative effects. Using protein and fat as your primary energy during ketosis, when you use ketone bodies for energy instead of sugar, can result in constipation and acidic breath. That's if you are a strict follower. In the desire to lose weight, most people are not bothered with those mild symptoms. But there are bigger issues. These types of diets can damage your cells and organs.

The Effect of Low-Carb Diets on Hormones

High-protein/low-carb diets are also bad for thyroid functions since excess protein prevents the thyroid hormone from converting to its active form. All the effects of your thyroid hormone come from the free hormone. As a result, a sluggish thyroid and a slower metabolism happens in some people. A high-fat diet shuts off human growth hormone or HGH, which also impairs cellular communication, one of the ten hallmarks of aging.

A low-carb diet will help you lose weight if that is your only goal. But those diets are not sustainable as a long-term eating plan. Any extreme diet that goes against the instinct of what your body needs is hard to maintain. But the biggest issue I have with high-protein/low-carb diets is that they are counterproductive when it comes to longevity. Too much protein produces higher levels of uric acid as a by-product, which can cause kidney stones and heart disease.

Low-Carb Diets and Cancer

When I did my media tour of *The Perfect 10 Diet*, I heard arguments from interviewers who said things like "I lost fifty pounds on this high-protein/low-carb diet; it has worked well for me, and I am not even hungry. My sugar is better, my diabetes has improved. How can you argue with these results,

Doc?" I had to educate the interviewers and I would say, "Oh yes, they are good in some ways, they are great for weight loss, but they have to be greatly modified by reducing the excess protein and eliminating all the chemicals." Sugar is not the only poison we have to avoid to be healthy. We have to avoid all chemicals.

But it's hard to change people's minds—especially when there are food industries built around a low-carb lifestyle, just like low-fat, but what I'm saying is the truth. I am not into quick fixes. I do not believe in superficial health tips that can endanger your health in the long term. I am not the kind of doctor who gives Band-Aid solutions with simple messages like "follow a low-carb diet."

Those simple messages are not enough to make you live longer. There are ten hallmarks of aging, and we have to target them all. But any health advice you implement from this book, even simple ones, can make an enormous difference in your life.

My advice? Choose natural food instead of a low-carb chocolate bar with soy protein isolate or protein shakes with artificial sweeteners and chemicals. You should have no desire to put any chemicals in your body.

Say no to bad types of protein on low-carb diets. Eating processed meats with added nitrites, like bacon, sausages, baloney, and Canadian bacon, can help you lose weight. But consuming nitrites in the long term is linked to increased cancer risk for the esophagus, stomach, colon, and prostate in countless research studies. Nitrites in processed meats damage your DNA. You must protect your DNA, not damage it. Chromosomal instability is one of the ten hallmarks of aging. If you like to eat bacon or sausage, go for the ones preserved with sea salt.

Apart from kidney stones and increased cancer risk, heart disease is another big issue with high-protein/low-carb diets. Heart disease is linked to eating too much protein—not to eating too much saturated fat. This is not a typo or a mistake. I will repeat myself. *Heart disease is a disease of eating too much protein, and not of eating too much saturated fat.*

The Link Between Low-Carb Diets and Heart Disease

When people go to the doctor worried about their hearts, they may get a calcium scan. It is a test that tells if there is arterial damage. But this test misses early damage. When calcium gets deposited in a plaque, it may be too late. This maladaptive repair happens when calcium gets deposited on top of cholesterol already inside the arteries.

At first, the expansion of a plaque is related to cholesterol being deposited in the outer arterial wall, but it eventually encroaches on the lumen. It's like a street getting blocked by parked cars. This is stenosis. At a certain point, the plaque gets calcified, or calcium gets deposited in it.

The body is trying to stop the damage, but here is the bad news. It is like a repair system after a major fire or flood that already happened inside a house: it is too late. The plaque may get detached, and you can suffer a heart attack. A CT angiogram can tell when the damage starts long before the calcium gets deposited, but it is not a standard test.

There are several ways high-protein diets may promote heart disease. When you eat certain proteins in high amounts, uric acid levels, a by-product, go up. And that's not good. High uric acid in the blood is linked to a higher mortality. It appears high uric acid leads to endothelial dysfunction through inflammation and oxidative stress. This leads to the formation of the unstable lipid plaque in your arteries, which eventually leads to heart attacks. Many people on low-carb diets have calcium deposits in the arteries after many years on these diets. This is indicative of cholesterol getting stuck in the arteries. High-protein/low-carb diet followers can develop hardening of the arteries by 30 percent more than dieters on a natural food program. Hardening of the arteries happens when calcium gets deposited in your supple arteries. Is that what you want?

Moreover, the plaque that builds up tends to be unstable, thinner, and breaks off more easily, increasing the risk of a blockage and heart attack. Colchicine, a drug that lowers inflammation, seems to prevent heart disease in new studies. This medication has not been widely adopted by cardiologists, yet it offers more superior protection than statins. In 2023, colchicine was approved by the FDA to prevent heart attacks as it reduces the incidence of heart attacks by a whopping 30 percent.

Another reason for the increased risk with low-carb diets is that excess protein also breaks down to a protein called homocysteine, which makes the cholesterol stickier. More cholesterol gets deposited in the arteries. Low-carb diets also negatively impact the hallmarks of aging.

Effect of Low-Carb Diets on the Hallmarks of Aging

Excess protein also activates the mTOR pathway. When mTOR becomes active, it sends a signal to macrophages to grow bigger than necessary to clean the plaque. As I said earlier, mTOR pathway is the elevator in the hotel that you do not want to overload or overuse when you get older. If this pathway is overloaded, overused, or overactivated, the whole hotel or the building will come crumbling down. In plain English, you will have a shorter life! Please do not fall for this 200-year-old approach.

Keto Diets

In the 2020s, keto diets became all the craze as they displaced the use of the term low-carb. It is the same concept but with a twist. Pick up any magazine, and you will find the newest keto diet on the market. But those keto diets are nothing but a recycled old idea from the 1920s. Back then, fasting was a way to treat epilepsy. The theory was that if you eliminate carbs, it will cause ketosis, with the body using ketone bodies instead of sugar for its nutritional needs.

In 1924, Dr. Russel Wilder at the Mayo Clinic named it the ketogenic diet. The name stuck. Somehow, a hundred years later, keto diets are back and are all the rage! There are three types of keto diets: standard, cyclical, and targeted. Each one focuses on a dieter's goals with varying percentages of fat, protein, and carbs in each version. The concept here is to use fat as the primary source of energy. You reduce carbs drastically and increase fats to a whopping 70 percent! Again, a very-high-fat diet negatively affects the secretion of human growth hormone, or HGH. That is the last thing you want to do if you want to age gracefully.

You run the same risk as high-protein/low-carb when you consume too much protein (25 percent). Again, high protein even at 25 percent negatively impairs the mTOR pathway. You want to use this pathway less when you age, or your risk of death goes up. Uric acid levels go up too. I just talked about that.

The danger does not stop here. High-fat diets turn off sirtuins. Sirtuins are the CEO of the cells that you want activated to clean up cell debris and old cells, not to shut them off! You will also miss the good nutrients found in good carbs that can help your stem cells and turn on your sirtuins.

Eating red meat and processed meats are not keys to longevity. How can a salad made of lettuce, bacon bits, and tons of cheese deliver to your body a good amount of healthy nutrients?

I do like, however, a certain aspect of keto diets that can be used in one meal only, such as eating a fat-rich breakfast like eggs and cheese or drinking a keto coffee (coffee made with butter) in the morning to shut down hunger on the days of intermittent fasting. Dave Asprey, a biohacker and a lifestyle guru, invented this keto coffee. But the keto lifestyle should not be a short- or long-term eating plan. You will learn about intermittent fasting in Chapter 14.

Popular Diets with Packaged Foods

Often these popular diets feature prepackaged foods. The food is sometimes even delivered right to your front door. This means you don't have to calculate the vitamins, proteins, and other nutrients in the food because the company says they are offering a "proper and balanced diet." But this often isn't true.

Many nutrients are lost in these packaged foods that have been frozen for months. Many ingredients in processed and packaged foods are toxic, especially when you eat them in substantial amounts since they contain vegetable oils that are manufactured fats. Corn, cottonseed, and soybean oils are often found in those packaged and frozen foods. These oils are highly processed, and the extraction method involves using toxic chemicals, such as hexane, that can alter your genome.

Processed and packaged foods are high in omega-6 fats, which promote inflammation when eaten in large amounts. A diet high in vegetable oils, which all contain omega-6 in excess, is linked to many types of cancer. Those oils are cancer-promoting when heated once that package is microwaved. These types of man-made oils have no place in a healthy diet.

Another dangerous substance, bisphenol A (BPA), is in the packaging of the plastic containers and beverages, including water, used for these meals. This chemical has been used to make certain plastics and resins since the 1950s. It is a polycarbonate, a synthetic resin. BPA leaches out of the plastic and into the food. In the body, BPA disrupts hormone production. High BPA is linked to insulin resistance, diabetes, and obesity. These chemicals are hormone disruptors that slow down your metabolism. When you go off these diets, you'll gain the weight back; this leads to yo-yo dieting, which is frustrating and ineffective.

Choose Natural Foods and a Balanced Diet

Natural food and a clean, balanced diet are essential for your body's best performance—not chemicals. All these diets not only negatively affect the ten hallmarks of aging but they also affect all our health negatively. Changing people's minds about this type of dieting isn't easy. We all have been brainwashed about what is healthy.

The way I see it, you should treat your body better than a $3 million Bugatti. A Bugatti needs more than gasoline to run. It needs frequent oil changes, a charged battery, brake fluid, windshield-wiper fluid, air in the tires, and everything else most cars need. But what it needs the most is clean, premium, non-degraded gasoline without any harmful additives. The same goes for your body. It needs balanced, natural, high-quality food for the best performance. What you put in your body makes a world of difference in what you will achieve.

A Patient's Story

When Anna first came to see me, she was incredibly frustrated with her weight. She was forty-two years old and had been overweight since she was a teen. She had recently gone up to 180 pounds and had been put on cholesterol and blood pressure drugs. She could not understand how this was possible when she carefully followed a low-carb diet. She did lose some weight but reached a plateau. I explained why a balanced diet was better for her health.

Together, we worked on improving her diet. She started to consume more fiber-rich vegetables and cut down on low-carb chocolate bars, which had more calories than fruits. For breakfast, she replaced eggs with bacon to eggs on whole wheat toast. She started snacking on hummus and lettuce instead of protein shakes. Anna lost thirty pounds in one year. She was able to get off her cholesterol and blood pressure drugs and has never felt better.

Remember . . .

- All four concepts of popular diets negatively affect the hallmarks of aging, so get off them.
- Low-fat diets were invented by politicians, not scientists.
- Low-fat diets mess up many hormones.
- Low-carb followers can develop hardening of the arteries in a few years after being on those diets.
- Do not eat low-fat products; they are full of sugar.
- Do not eat low-carb products; they are full of chemicals.
- Stay away from all refined vegetable oils.
- Keto diets are a new twist on the low-carb concept.
- Do not fear full-fat dairy products, including milk and butter.
- If you must eat processed food, read labels to see which fats and which chemicals were added. Choose wisely.
- Always avoid all processed meats and smoked meats. They damage your DNA and can lead to cancer.
- Eat a lot of fresh, preferably organic, vegetables and fruits.

PART III

The Ageless Revolution Plan: Principles of the Ageless Diet, Superfoods, Spices, and Longevity

CHAPTER 9

The Ageless Diet

It's easy to stand in the crowd
but it takes courage to stand alone.
—Mahatma Gandhi

When I authored *The Perfect 10 Diet*, my message was simple: follow a balanced and natural diet that is good for your hormones. As you've learned, thanks to low-fat diets, we are eating more sugar and refined carbohydrates. This spikes insulin, the fat-storing hormone, and making us hungrier.

Compared to the 1970s, most people are eating an extra 400 calories a day! No wonder obesity is rampant in our society. Globally, about 12 percent of all cancers are related to obesity. *The Ageless Revolution* is not a diet book; it is a plan for longevity. You can't live longer if you don't eat right. Obesity can reduce your lifespan by years, if not decades. It puts you at risk also for heart disease, type 2 diabetes, and stroke. If you need detailed advice on how to lose weight or how to follow a balanced natural diet, consult with a nutritionist who supports the research I advocate, or read my previous book, *The Perfect 10 Diet: 10 Key Hormones That Hold the Secret to Losing Weight and Feeling Great Fast.* The Perfect 10 Diet balances ten key hormones, so it optimizes your metabolism. The Perfect 10 Diet does not interfere with insulin, leptin, human growth hormone, or the sex hormones. These hormones play a major role in weight loss as they control your metabolism.

Introducing The Ageless Diet

The Ageless Diet (my new and improved Perfect 10 Diet) is hugely different from low-fat, low-carb, keto, and other diets since it helps balance hormones and does not interfere with their functioning. Hormonal balance is essential for cells to communicate, which is important for longevity. Cellular communication is optimized when you eat natural food. You also improve your health by eating superfoods. But, first, let's learn about what macronutrients are. Most importantly, this diet is good for the hallmarks of aging.

The Macronutrients

Our macronutrients come from three sources: carbohydrates, protein, and fats.

1. Carbohydrates are found in vegetables, fruits, beans, and whole grains.
2. Protein is found in eggs, seafood, poultry, beans, mushrooms, and nuts. It is also in beef, pork, and lamb.
3. Fats are divided into three different subgroups:
   - Saturated fats are solid at room temperature and with refrigeration. They are found in butter, coconut, cocoa butter, dairy, ghee, and palm oil.
   - Monounsaturated fats are liquid at room temperature but turn solid with refrigeration. Monounsaturated fats are found in avocados, nuts, olive oil, grapeseed oil, and animal fat.
   - Polyunsaturated oils are liquid at room temperature and with refrigeration. They are further divided into two subgroups:
     A. Omega-3 fatty acids are found in fish and flaxseed oil.
     B. Omega-6 fatty acids are found in peanuts and corn. They are also found in man-made fats such as cottonseed and soybean oils.

Bad Fats

As I discussed, bad fats are man-made. Vegetable oils (corn, soybean, cottonseed) are processed with chemicals during the extraction process. They damage the cell walls when heated with free electrons. To make matters worse, trans fats are plastic fats that are formed when vegetable oils (soybean, corn oil, or others) undergo a process called hydrogenation or partial hydrogenation. Both processes add a hydrogen atom to the oil under pressure to make the oil more stable, or to make solid fats, like margarine such as I Can't Believe It's Not Butter. Again, these bad fats and trans fats should never be part of your diet.

Omega-7

Most people are not aware of omega-7s, but these fats provide unique health effects. Omega-7 can reduce the risk of type 2 diabetes, prevent the buildup of atherosclerotic plaque, increase beneficial HDL, and lower an inflammation marker called *C-reactive protein*, which is associated with an increased risk for heart attack and stroke. This newly discovered fat molecule is so important that Harvard Medical School has applied for a patent on it. You can find omega-7 in macadamia nuts and macadamia oils.

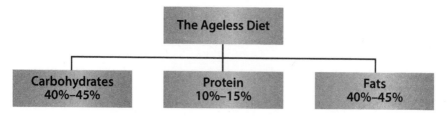

Percentage of macronutrients on The Ageless Diet.

The Ageless Diet

The amount of animal protein in your diet should be 10 to 15 percent. If you're involved in anaerobic activities such as lifting weights, you need more. Carbs and fats are in equal amounts at 40 to 45 percent.

As you age, you may increase protein to 20 percent starting from age thirty, so you do not lose muscle mass. But protein should not be used as your main source of energy at 50 percent like in low-carb diets because it's not a clean source. This increases uric acid. Excess protein also overloads the mTOR pathway, one of the nutrient-sensing pathways.

How Do I Calculate My Daily Protein Intake?

The palm of your hand is about 3 ounces. That is about 85 grams. It can give you a guide on how much protein to eat in a day. Your body needs 0.8–1 gram per kilogram. Divide your weight in pounds by 2.2 to get your body weight in kilograms. Let us say, for example, you are 160 pounds. Divide your weight by 2.2, you get 72.72 kilograms. You need to eat 72 grams of protein a day, or the size of your palm. Most athletes need about 2.2 grams of protein per kilogram of body weight per day. So double that amount of protein you eat in a day if you work out and lift weights. You will need the extra protein for muscle buildup and repair.

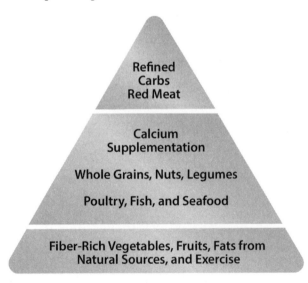

The Ageless Diet food and activity pyramid.

Level 1—the base. The base is anchored by fiber-rich vegetables and natural fats that balance hormones. Think of this as the foundation of your diet. Do not fear natural fats; instead, eat two to three servings a day. Choose, for instance, adding half an avocado and some olive oil on your salad. This fat will make you feel full, and you will eat less. Eat one to two servings of fruit daily. Excess fructose, even if it is natural, is bad for our bodies. The body can only manage 25 to 40 grams of fructose a day. Fructose is mostly used by the liver cells. Excess fructose can cause a fatty liver. Again, do not consume any manufactured or refined vegetable oils.

Eat at least seven to nine vegetables with assorted colors every day. Think of broccoli, cauliflower, and spinach. These vegetables are full of super nutrients. Add lots of spices to your meals such as turmeric, saffron, and ginger. The base level includes exercise because anaerobic exercise is essential to boost human growth hormone (HGH) production, which can keep you lean and fit. Exercise also activates your sirtuins and invigorates your cells.

Level 2—the middle. Eat one to three servings of protein a day. A serving is the size of the palm of your hand. You can eat three servings of protein if you work out and lift weights or after age thirty when muscle loss starts to increase at a rate of 3 to 5 percent per decade. Preferred sources of protein are eggs, mushrooms, beans, organic poultry, and seafood. When it comes to longevity, the less animal protein you eat, the better. Go for more vegetarian sources such as beans.

Eat whole grains in moderation. Whole grains can support your hormones and fill you up. Reduce grains if you need to lose weight. Some wild rice is okay. Even better, have cauliflower rice—not rice in the traditional sense, but a great substitute. Brown rice is a little better than white rice for its effect on blood sugar levels, but it is still bad in excess. That's because brown rice contains an antinutrient called phytic acid, which reduces the body's ability to absorb iron and zinc when eaten in excess. Soaking the rice before cooking can help retain some of the nutritional value. You can have a tennis-ball-size scoop of whole wheat pasta for lunch, or a slice of whole-grain toast with your eggs for breakfast.

Eat legumes such as lentils, peas, chickpeas, and black beans. Have unsalted nuts such as macadamia nuts and almonds (a handful two to four times a week). Dairy should be limited. If you consume dairy, go for full-fat, not the fat-free variety. Go organic if you can afford it. Have almond milk, coconut milk, or cashew milk instead. Calcium supplementation is better than dairy consumption. Milk has excess calories, which are not needed as you embark on this journey. Excess dairy has been linked to prostate cancer in men. If you consume dairy, limit the amount to eight ounces. That's the size of a small cup from Starbucks.

Level 3—the top. Refined carbs spike insulin, so they are at the top of the pyramid and should be limited or, if possible, excluded from your diet. Having a cookie should only be an occasional treat, not the basis of a healthy diet. Sharing a dessert with friends at a restaurant occasionally is okay as long as you don't overdo it.

Pasta, cereals, candy, white rice, and sweets should be greatly limited or excluded since they are converted to glucose quickly in your body and raise blood sugar levels. Avoid foods that contain nitrites like bacon, baloney, Canadian bacon, ham, luncheon meats, and sausages. Smoked foods contain chemicals and carcinogens too. If you eat processed meats, choose the sea-salt-preserved variety. Limit red meat, beef, pork, or lamb to three to six ounces every two to three weeks. Avoid grilling meat. Red grilled meat has been linked to colon cancer since heterocyclic amines are formed. Heterocyclic amines are chemical compounds that form when meat is grilled and act like carcinogens. Instead, have red meat as part of a stew or in soups.

The Ageless Diet: Snacks

Snacks are optional on the Ageless Diet. You can have one to two snacks a day on the days you work out or if you are hungry. Frequent eating and snacks inhibit sirtuins, which need to be activated to clean cells from debris. Snacks are ideal for people who suffer from hypoglycemia or low sugar, and for folks who work out regularly.

Avoid Fried Foods

It goes without saying that fried food, especially from fast-food restaurants, is not good for longevity. If you like the taste and texture of fried food, invest in an air fryer. It can give you the crunch without the added calories. Use no oils or minimal amounts. If you do, use a high-burning oil such as grapeseed or macadamia oils.

How the Ageless Diet Differs from the Popular Concepts

As you can see, the Ageless Diet is vastly different from all popular diets as it is balanced. It aims to support hormones and does not mess them up. It eliminates all chemicals and processed food. In addition, a balanced diet with lots of superfoods and an abundance of spices will give you an edge on longevity. I realize that ordering eggs with fruit for breakfast may not be the norm. But following the low-carb approach of "bacon and eggs but hold the bread" means you are already starting your day with a poor meal choice. If great health is your goal, you must consider what you are putting in your mouth and body. It takes some effort, but it is certainly doable.

You can control the foods you consume by eating more often at home, and you also save money! Remember, the rewards are huge: a healthier and longer life. You can prevent disease and even reverse the damage of unhealthy diets and bad lifestyle habits.

The Ageless Revolution and Losing Weight

When you follow a balanced diet, you stabilize your blood sugar level and balance your hormones, so your cells can communicate effectively. Now hormones can enter the cells, and this helps you lose weight. Eating whole foods and natural fats in moderation also helps you feel full, which can help you avoid overeating and thus lose weight. As you incorporate natural fats into your diet such as avocados, butter, and olive oil you will also lose weight by lowering insulin, promoting satiety, and feeling full. When you eliminate excess calories from sugar, you'll also lose weight because of your balanced hormones.

Tips on Losing Weight on *The Ageless Revolution*

Being overweight predisposes you to a variety of illnesses, including early heart disease, cancer, and type 2 diabetes.

1. Eat a little natural fat with each meal. This helps to shut down hunger. Have a slice of cheese with your eggs. Add olive oil to your salads.

2. Spread a teaspoon of butter or macadamia butter on your whole wheat toast instead of jelly.

3. Toss a few thin slices of avocado or nuts on your salad. Natural fats provide you with satiety. Fats will be just one trick up your sleeve.

4. Eat vegetables first. Often, when people to go restaurants, they start with the white bread. This spikes insulin, the fat-storing hormone, and causes hunger. Instead, start with your vegetables or a salad before you eat protein. This will reduce the amount of insulin going in your bloodstream, so you will be less hungry to go for the bread or dessert.

5. Choose alcoholic drinks that are low in sugar: a glass of red wine or rosé.

6. Eat slowly. Chew and savor your food.

7. Drink plenty of ice water. Ice water helps burn calories as your body will have to warm it up for absorption.

8. If you eat dessert, go for a choice that is healthy, like fruit and cheese. If it is a rich, sugary dessert, do so only occasionally, and share with your party.

The Perfect 10 Diet Versus the Ageless Diet

The *Perfect 10 Diet* was written in 2010 with the goal to lose weight and achieve great health. If you need to lose weight, you will need a solid weight-loss program. This is beyond the scope of this book. Again, read *The Perfect 10 Diet*. The Ageless Diet aims to clean your body from all chemicals. It may help with weight loss but isn't particularly designed for that goal. I must address and clarify two things in *The Perfect 10 Diet*. I advised using agave as a sweetener in *The Perfect 10 Diet*. If you consume agave, it should be from the plant itself, and it should not be refined. And there is a max amount. Again, the body can manage 25 to 40 grams of fructose a day. Excess fructose is bad. One thing's for sure: fructose is better than artificial sweeteners. Also, soy is not linked to breast cancer, but eating substantial amounts of soy can lead to an underactive thyroid. So I still see soy as a moderately favorable source of protein. It has been a few years since I have written *The Perfect 10 Diet*, and new research comes every day. But *The Perfect 10 Diet* is as solid now as it was fourteen years ago. I still stand with everything I advocated years ago.

What You Need to Know About Water

Your body can't function without water. We need it to hydrate our cells and our body, to keep our bodies from overheating, and to carry all the nutrients and minerals we need for cellular health and regeneration to the right places. When you exercise, drinking water improves oxygen intake and transports it to your brain and other cell tissues.

How Much Water Should You Drink?

In the United States, the goal is to consume eight 8-ounce cups of water per day or 64 ounces of liquid. How much you need to drink depends on who you are. A 210-pound man needs more water than a 105-pound woman. The U.S. National Academies of Sciences, Engineering, and Medicine says, "Your bodies are not the same, so your hydration requirements are not the same."

Their recommendation, widely used as a standard in scientific communities, is that men consume 15.5 cups (124 ounces) of water per day, and women consume 11.5 cups (92 ounces) of water. Remember that 20 percent of the water you take in is through food, so you can safely say that men must drink twelve cups of water and women should drink nine cups of water.

Even those numbers will fluctuate based on how much you are exercising, whether you live in a hot environment, whether you are ill or pregnant, how much you sweat, how much water you exhale, and how much water your body might need when it is unusually stressed. In fact, you may need to increase this amount of water by 20 percent if you start to do intermittent fasting, as food contains water too. Bottom line, make sure you are always hydrated.

What Kind of Water Is Best to Consume?

It is important to drink clean, filtered water in adequate amounts for your body size and to replenish what you lose through sweat. Preferably water from natural sources: mineral, iceberg, glacier, and especially spring water. Flavored mineral, seltzer, filtered, and even tap water will hydrate you. Add lemon or some fruit to add some taste.

The only fixed rule is to avoid drinking sugary beverages and any liquids laden with sweeteners, preservatives, or chemicals like those in many sodas—especially the diet versions, which may include aspartame, ammonia, citric acid, and potassium benzoate. Soda also leaches calcium out of the bones.

Fluoride, which is present in most U.S. tap water, can be harmful. Whoever thought of that idea? Depending on your sensitivity, tap water can cause hypothyroidism, and even the complete cessation of thyroid function in some folks. Also, fluoride can damage your pineal gland, which regulates control of the circadian cycle of sleep and makes melatonin, which is essential to keep your mitochondria intact. Mitochondrial dysfunction is one of the ten hallmarks of aging.

Alkaline Versus Regular Water

There is a trend now to favor alkaline water over regular water. Alkaline water has a higher pH level (potential of hydrogen) of about nine, whereas regular water has a pH of 7.4. Some researchers claim that alkaline water has anti-aging benefits and helps fight cancer. It is not known currently if this is true. However, although alkaline water is more expensive, drinking it can keep you more hydrated than regular water.

To save money on *The Ageless Revolution,* you can make your own alkaline water at home by adding a half teaspoon of baking soda to 8 ounces of water. Or buy retail pH drops or a water filter with alkaline pods.

Another caveat: do not use plastic bottles. Your endocrine system can be affected by bisphenol A (BPA) found in plastic water bottles, a hormone disruptor. It's also not ecologically smart to use plastic. Bottled water comes in a variety of natural flavors, so there is something for everyone; even coffee and tea drinkers benefit as it is untrue that those drinks' diuretic effects exceed their ability to hydrate.

A Patient's Story

Carly is one of my patients who is in her forties. Ever since high school, she has been battling her weight but had no success. Carly started dieting at age eighteen, and for years she was a yo-yo dieter. Nothing worked. She estimates she has been on every diet on the planet but has had a steady weight at 200 pounds for years. During the Covid-19 pandemic, she gained another 80 pounds, and her weight ballooned to 280 pounds.

After falling in her apartment, she tore the ACL in her left knee and had to use a wheelchair. She was shocked when her orthopedic surgeon told her she was too heavy to withstand surgery. But this was a wake-up call for Carly. I placed Carly on the Ageless Diet, which emphasizes vegetables and low-sugar fruits, seafood, beans, and whole grains. She allowed herself a dark piece of chocolate every few days. Carly lost 120 pounds in two years and did not need knee surgery as her new MRI shows.

A balanced diet is essential for your longevity. Stay away from fad diets as you embark on this new journey. You alone hold the keys to your lifespan.

Remember . . .

- Follow a natural, balanced diet.

- Eat fewer animal products.

- Stay away from fad diets.

- Eat more poultry, beans, seafood, and mushrooms.

- Stay away from sugar and refined carbs.

- Avoid refined vegetable oils and trans fats.

- The palm of your hand can be your guide to knowing how much protein you need to eat every day.

- Double your protein intake if you work out.

- At restaurants, eat your vegetables first before any bread or protein.

- Drink a lot of water (at least sixty-four ounces) and adjust that amount depending on your activity, the weather, and your health. Men and women need different amounts.

- Use the food choices and food plan lists in the Appendix.

CHAPTER 10

Top Anti-Aging Foods and Beverages

*The doctor of the future will no longer treat
the human frame with drugs, but rather will cure
and prevent disease with nutrition.*
—Thomas Edison

Today, 90 percent of the United State's $4.1 trillion spent in health care is on is lifestyle preventable chronic diseases: heart disease, cancer, diabetes, and dementia. During the Covid-19 pandemic, more than 60 percent of the hospitalizations could have been prevented if we were on the right track. Those who were mostly affected by Covid-19 were the obese, elderly, and people with high blood pressure. It is time to change our doomed path. Joel Osteen dubs it "Second Chance." *The Ageless Revolution* is your second chance to change your genetic destiny. It is a chance to age differently. So forget low-fat, low-carb, and keto, and look forward to a bright future. In *The Ageless Revolution*, you do not need to be rich to follow its affordable principles. There is no need to eat expensive, hard-to-find food options. You just need to eat clean; it's that simple. People in Costa Rica and Ikaria cracked the longevity code with little to no money. You can follow in their footsteps too.

You've learned about the habits and practices of people who live in the five Blue Zones and beyond. Now, it's time to put all this information into action. Forget about your salad made of lettuce, croutons, bacon bits, and low-fat dressing made with soybean oil that you thought was healthy. You need a different eating model. A balanced diet with lots of superfoods. Welcome to *The Ageless Revolution.*

To have longevity, you need lots of foods that deliver superior nutrients with anti-aging benefits. So go for vegetables with various colors: blue, orange, red, pink, and yellow. In other words, go for superfoods. Why? Super nutrients. Any car can run on regular gasoline, but premium gasoline is the best for performance. Just like a car, you cannot put contaminants into your body and think your body can work just fine. Instead, your performance will suffer, or your body will suddenly break down on the road of life.

So don't bog down your body with junk like sugar, chemicals, and manufactured fats. Just like a car engine must be clean and well oiled, your body must be properly maintained with top anti-aging foods. Take care of your body, and it will serve you well. This means learning and thinking about the foods you are eating and understanding whether it is good or bad for your body. Remember, knowledge is power. Now let us look at those terrific top anti-aging foods that will keep your biological engine running smoothly for life.

Berries

Berries are not only one of the healthiest foods in the world but they are also superfoods. Berries are loaded with antioxidants, which help keep free radicals at bay. Free radicals damage cell walls, causing oxidative stress and impaired cell communication, which is one of the ten hallmarks of aging. Berries are rich in resveratrol, which activate sirtuins too.

Acai berries, which come from Brazil, have the highest concentration of antioxidants of all berries, but blueberries, blackberries, and raspberries are also chock-full of antioxidants. Berries have a minimal impact on blood-sugar levels and are tasty, very low in calories, and filling. They're also high in fiber and help fight inflammation.

Eat berries often. Have them on the side with eggs for breakfast. Have them as a snack with some unsweetened whipped cream. Throw a few berries on your salad instead of croutons or bacon bits. Eat these superfoods often for great health and longevity.

Fish

Fish is not just protein rich; it is also rich in the omega-3 fatty acids that help prevent cholesterol buildup in your arteries, high blood pressure, and heart-related plaques. Omega-3 fatty acids also help reduce inflammation that happens with aging cell accumulation, one of the ten hallmarks of aging. Fish supports the stem cells. Remember Plastic Man in Chapter 3, who can become anything you want him to be. Fish is also brain food. The highest amount of omega-3 is found in salmon, tuna steaks, mackerel, herring, trout, anchovies, and sardines. Eat fish and other seafood a few times a week.

Eat Fish Lower on the Food Chain

High-food-chain fish are usually bigger, predatory, and have more mercury because of biomagnification. This includes sharks and swordfish. Mercury can impair brain functions. Mercury also impairs your DNA.

Fish and other seafood with lower mercury content include whitefish, pollock, herring, sardines, char, hake, blue crab, shrimp, clams, mussels, and oysters. Salmon is immensely popular but make sure your salmon is wild caught not farm raised. Farm-raised salmon and other fish spend their lives in dirty vats, and they are fed processed food to plump them up. They are also fed antibiotics, fungicides, and herbicides.

Farmed salmon has been found to contain toxic chemicals such as methylmercury and dioxins. As if that was not bad enough, PCBs (polychlorinated biphenyls), chemical waste from industrial processes, found in farmed salmon were eight times higher than those found in wild salmon. Again, all those chemicals are bad for your DNA. Go wild!

Whitefish is a term that refers to fish such as cod, whiting, rockfish, and tilapia. Most fish that are low in mercury live near or on the seafloor. Their flesh is white and rich in proteins, fats, sodium, potassium, vitamins, selenium, magnesium, and calcium. When eating cod, make sure you are careful about where the fish comes from. Schools of Atlantic cod are growing scarce, so avoid it. Look for Alaskan cod, which is abundant, well managed, and more often wild caught.

Eggs

For decades, we were told to avoid egg yolks and to go for egg whites instead. This was bad advice. Eggs are a top superfood and a reliable source of protein and good fats. It's no mistake that eggs are eaten frequently in all of the Blue Zones. The B vitamins in eggs help reduce brain inflammation and prevent Alzheimer's disease. The yolk has nutrients that help prevent macular degeneration, the leading cause of blindness in the elderly. Have eggs for breakfast a few times a week, and do not fear the cholesterol found in them. Go for pasture-fed or organic eggs because those contain omega-3 fatty acids. Avoid egg beaters, which contain added chemicals.

Fermented Products

Gut health matters when it comes to longevity. If your gut is unhealthy, you cannot absorb food or nutrients. Fermented products like sauerkraut, kimchi, and plain yogurt improve your gut flora or bacteria. They are also great sources of vitamin D, protein, and calcium, which are important for having strong bones.

Plain full-fat yogurt contains live cultures called probiotics, or healthy bacteria, which prevent the growth of unhealthy bacteria in your gut. Look for *live bacteria* labels on yogurt because pasteurization kills the healthy bacteria in yogurt. Kefir, especially from organic sources, is nine times richer in probiotics than yogurt. Kefir can make an excellent choice for breakfast or a quick snack. Allergic to dairy? Try some Kombucha. Support your gut health in every way you can.

Avocados

Avocados are fruits with "good fat." They help the absorption of fat-soluble nutrients like vitamins A, D, K, and E and also contain fiber and potassium. The carotenoids found in avocados can help eye health, and vitamin-E oxidants protect from tissue damage as well as strengthen the immune system. Snack on half an avocado occasionally or toss some avocado pieces on your salad.

Cruciferous Vegetables

You do not need a doctor to tell you vegetables are great for your health, but cruciferous vegetables are the *best* vegetables you can eat. Cruciferous vegetables include Brussels sprouts, broccoli, cabbage, cauliflower, collard greens, kale, mustard greens, radishes, and turnips. They are a major source of fiber, vitamins, and phytochemicals that can offer protection against many types of cancer. Cruciferous vegetables help with estrogen metabolism. Next time you eat a salad, choose kale as the base instead of romaine lettuce. Make sure to eat at least three cruciferous vegetables a week. Eat cruciferous vegetables raw or cooked. You'll find a delicious cauliflower cream soup recipe in the recipe section. Try it. You'll love it.

Green Tomatoes

Green tomatoes are unripe tomatoes. There are also heirloom tomatoes that are green when ripe. Tomatidine, a compound found in green tomatoes, was found to extend lifespan in animal models and human cells. This compound influences the action of mitochondria. By recycling slower-working mitochondria through a process called mitophagy, cells can improve efficiency. This means it helps get rid of the old and nonfunctioning mitochondria.

The National Institute of Aging found that worms given tomatidine lived longer because it reduced cellular aging. Researchers also found it slowed aging in human cells. Look for green tomatoes the next time you are in the supermarket, which add variety to your salads.

Dark Chocolate

Yes, dark chocolate is a superfood. It contains more cocoa, which has anti-aging benefits, than milk chocolate. Cocoa relaxes your arteries and reduces blood pressure.

Dark chocolate is also rich in antioxidants and flavonoids that help support healthy blood vessels and lower the risk of type 2 diabetes and dementia. Dark chocolate helps your stem cells stay alive longer. Have a piece of dark chocolate with a cup of herbal or black tea for your next snack. That will provide your body with mega-doses of antioxidants, especially those that fight inflammation—again, one of the ten hallmarks of aging. Always look for dark chocolate with at least 70 to 80 percent cocoa, made with cocoa butter, not with hydrogenated soybean oil.

Nuts

Eat nuts and live longer. Macadamia nuts, walnuts, almonds, pecans, pistachios, cashews, and Brazil nuts are all a reliable source of plant proteins that contain vitamins, minerals, and other phytochemicals, including antioxidants. They are rich in omega-3 fatty acids, calcium, nutrients to protect against heart disease, and much more.

Brazil nuts, a seed, are full of copper, niacin, vitamin E, magnesium, selenium, and fiber. Cashews, also a seed, fight type 2 diabetes. Pistachios are rich in lutein, which is good for your eyes and prevents macular degeneration. Pecans have twenty-plus vitamins and minerals and can significantly lower cholesterol. Walnuts can improve cognitive health, as well as protect and enhance skin and bone health.

Nuts' benefits include defense against premature aging. They can prevent liver and heart disease, and they may be able to fight breast cancer too. Eat a handful of nuts at least three to four times a week. You can add seven to ten years to your life by adding nuts to your diet. Now, that is longevity!

Whole Grains

Both the low-carb and keto craze made people eliminate bread and rice from their diets. But whole grains are good for us and help our stem cells. Whole grains include all three parts of the kernel: bran—the hard outer shell full of fiber, minerals, and antioxidants; endosperm—the middle section, which is mostly carbohydrates; and germ—the inner part packed with vitamins, minerals, proteins, and plant compounds.

The most accessible whole grains include wheat berries, oatmeal, millet, quinoa, brown rice, barley, buckwheat, bulgur, wild rice, and whole rye. Wheat bread is the most popular, but make sure "100 percent whole wheat flour" is listed in the ingredients. When it comes to brown rice, have it in lesser amounts.

Whole grains can lower the risk of cardiovascular disease, stroke, and type 2 diabetes. There is no reason to go low-carb, keto, and avoid bread all your life for longevity. You can still be thin and healthy while enjoying whole-wheat grains. Whole grains constitute 47 percent of the Sardinian diet. You do not have to go to that extreme.

Beans

We talked about how not all protein is created equal for longevity. Plant sources of protein like beans are healthier options than animal sources. Beans are a good source of fiber and folate and are low in calories. They encourage the growth of healthy gut bacteria and prevent gut disease. Gut health is one of the ten hallmarks of aging. Beans can help lower cholesterol and blood pressure and balance sugar levels. Antioxidants in beans tackle free radicals to boost the immune system, support heart health, and help prevent cancer. Add all kinds to your shopping list: lima beans, peas, kidney beans, black-eyed peas, garbanzo beans, red beans, white beans, black beans, navy beans—and any other beans that come to mind. Eat beans two to three times a week.

Limit soybeans because of their negative effect on thyroid health especially in women and children. If you eat soy, do so in moderation, once or twice a week. Soy in excess is also bad for testosterone in men.

Butter

Who would have thought that butter, which was vilified as an atherogenic fat for decades by the medical establishment, is now a top superfood! When I was a guest on *The View,* Whoopi Goldberg asked me, "Is butter healthy?" My answer was simple: Look at the longevity of the French, known as the French paradox. The French suffer few heart attacks while enjoying dishes and creamy sauces rich in butter. The French even live longer than we do here in the United States by eight to nine years.

Organic butter supplies vitamins A, D, E, K, beta carotene, omega-3 fatty acids, calcium, copper, chromium, manganese, and selenium. All these nutrients contribute to lowering cancer risk and preventing night blindness, vision loss, macular degeneration, and brittle bones. Butter helps reduce inflammation and UV damage to the skin, heal skin wounds, regulate hormone and thyroid functions, increase nutrients absorption, and boost antioxidants. Phew—that is a lot of benefits!

Saturated fats like those found in butter are considered bad by the medical establishment, but they are not. That is flawed research sponsored by the soybean lobby to promote their man-made refined vegetable oils. Lauric acid in butter has antibacterial, antifungal, antiviral, and anticancer properties.

Buy organic butter from grass-fed cows, rather than grain-fed cows, for a greater amount of heart-healthy nutrients, and use butter for all your cooking. Spread it on a piece of whole wheat toast for a great-tasting addition to your breakfast.

When I talked favorably about butter years ago on television, I was one of the first doctors to espouse this unorthodox view. Most doctors viewed butter as atherogenic. Today, I am glad to see butter now presented as a top-notch superfood on many TV shows. We are finally heading in the right direction.

Extra-Virgin Olive Oil

Extra-virgin olive oil is the unsung hero in the longevity books. It is like the Beyoncé of healthy fats. It's loaded with antioxidants, which combat free radicals that damage cell walls. It is used in abundance in the Mediterranean region. Whether you are putting it on your salad or using it when sautéing some mushrooms, it should be in your arsenal of weapons against aging. A word of caution: Do not heat at high temperatures or use for baking. This can create free radicals at extreme high temperatures.

Monk Fruit

Monk fruit produces a natural sweetener that packs plenty of good things in a small drop of extract. It is 150 to 200 times sweeter than sugar, yet it has zero calories. Studies on mice show monk fruit lowers blood sugar levels and oxidative stress, which can lead to disease. It can increase good cholesterol, or HDL, has antioxidants and anti-inflammatory properties, which help prevent damage to DNA, and inhibits cancer cell growth.

Instead of sugar, you can use a drop or two of monk fruit extract in beverages, smoothies, sauces, and dressings. You can find monk fruit in liquid, granules, and powder forms in health food stores and online. Make sure your brand does not have added erythritol, which is linked to an increased risk for heart attacks.

Coconut

Coconut is also condemned as an atherogenic fat by the medical establishment, but again, this is false. In fact, coconut is eaten in abundance in many Asian countries with very low incidence of heart disease.

Coconut has a high content of medium-chain triglycerides (MCTs), which provide instant energy and promote fat loss in overweight people.

MCTs are unique because they are more easily digested and do not follow the same route through your system as other fats. Instead, they are absorbed directly from your intestines into your liver, and they provide a source of rapidly available energy for your body. Unlike other fats, MCTs are not stored by your body as fat.

Want to be in a state of ketosis to lose weight? You can do that by fasting for twelve hours or more. Or if this idea is unappealing or sounds too difficult, include more medium-chain triglycerides in your diet like those found in coconuts. The body uses these types of fats for energy and not storage.

Coconut is low in carbs, so it also has minimal impact on insulin levels. Coconut is rich in minerals and nutrients like manganese, which is essential for strong bones. Add coconut milk to your favorite dishes or eat coconut as a snack.

Bone Broth

For decades, the medical establishment advised us to make our soups with margarine and refined vegetable oils, but bone broth has been a staple for thousands of years and for good reason, it contains collagen. As we age, we lose collagen in our skin and joints. That's why dermatologists use fillers such as Radiesse for aging faces to stimulate collagen production. We need collagen more than ever—and we can get that extra collagen from bone broth.

Bone broth can be used as a base for soups and stews filled with vegetables, fish, or some meat, or eaten as it is. It's a clear, protein-rich liquid made by simmering meaty animal joints and bones in water. It increases plasma levels of health-promoting amino acids like glutamine and galantine, as well as glycine and proline, which create collagen.

Don't like soups? Eat the bone marrow. Don't like the rich taste? Take supplements. In trials, bone broth collagen supplements improved the hydration, elasticity, and appearance of wrinkles in the skin, and increased the bone mineral density in postmenopausal women. The collagen derived from chicken cartilage even decreases pain and stiffness and increases joint function in patients with osteoarthritis.

In addition, the amino acids such as glycine in bone broth support healthy sleep patterns, even in patients with insomnia. Glycine regulates our internal body clock and lowers body temperature as we prepare for sleep.

Galantine, the most abundant protein in bone broth, can be beneficial in tissue repair after injury and combined with vitamin C, it improves tendon repair and collagen synthesis after exercise. In the digestive tract, galantine binds with water to move food through the intestines, so it can be therapeutic for inflammatory bowel disease.

The amino acids found in bone broth can also protect the gut barrier. If this is damaged, it can disrupt immune function. The small intestine is the main site for nutrient absorption and the first line of defense in our immune system.

Citrus Fruits

Oranges and lemons have an interesting compound called hesperidin, which was first isolated in 1928 by a French chemist, M. Lebreton. It is in the fruit but mostly found in the white inner layer of citrus peels, which has anti-oxidant and anti-inflammatory properties. Hesperidin helps with high blood pressure, type 2 diabetes, and neurodegenerative disorders. It also helps with cognition and has anticancer properties.

Hesperidin also positively affects the AMPK pathway. This is the pathway that must be optimized as we age. It slows down as we age. So hesperidin acts like a mechanic to make sure the elevator for both carbs and protein is always working. The next time you make lemonade, use the whole lemon—not just the juice. Wash the lemon thoroughly and throw the whole lemon in the blender. This will give your lemonade a rich flavor and give you extra hesperidin to make you healthier. Go organic if you can to avoid pesticides. You can also take hesperidin as a supplement.

Sweet Purple Potatoes

Sweet purple potatoes may be the secret of longevity in Okinawa, in Japan. These potatoes are known for their anthocyanin content, natural pigments in the flesh and skin that give the tubers their purple hue. Anthocyanins have anti-inflammatory, antimicrobial, and antioxidant-like properties to protect the cells against the damage caused by free radicals and oxidative stress. This vegetable also supports healthy stem cells, which can serve many purposes in the body, depending on what's needed. Remember, stem cells are like Plastic Man, who can become anything you want him to be. Sweet purple potatoes vary in size and shape, depending on the variety and growing environment. Do not confuse sweet purple potatoes with red sweet potatoes, which are purple on the outside, white on the inside. Sweet purple potatoes look like regular white potatoes, but they are purple on the inside.

Sweet purple potatoes may be hard to find, so go to your local farmer's market or buy them online. They come in unique shades of saturated royal purples, violets, blue purple, dark purple, or almost black. Inside, the flesh is dense, starchy, and firm, with shades from solid purple to marbled purple, red, and white hues. Sweet purple potatoes were once known as the "food of the gods," and historically, they were reserved for Incan kings. They originated in South America and were brought to Japan in the 1600s.

Sweet purple potatoes have an earthy and nutty taste suited for cooked preparations such as roasting, boiling, baking, braising, mashing, grilling, and even pan-frying. It is important to note that the vibrant coloring will fade in the cooking process, but depending on the variety, the flesh will retain a light purple to lavender hue. Sweet purple potatoes can be used in any recipe calling for all-purpose, moderately starchy potatoes, and simmered into soups, curries, and stews. Delicious and healthy!

Mushrooms

Mushrooms are fungus and a good source of protein. Mushrooms are good for your immune system and good for gut health. Mushrooms contain prebiotics, which help in the growth of beneficial gut bacteria, which keeps your GI tract healthy and your immune system strong. Gut health is one of the ten hallmarks of aging.

Mushrooms also lower blood pressure and improve heart health and brain health. Try mushroom soup—it is so rich in taste. Or toss some mushrooms on your salad instead of croutons.

Tea

In the Blue Zones, tea drinking is popular, so I'd like to encourage you to cut back on coffee and follow in their footsteps. At the supermarket, you will find a variety of teas. It can get overwhelming. Each type of tea has its unique benefits. Purists consider only green tea, black tea, white tea, oolong tea, and pu-erh (a variety of fermented tea from China) as the real thing. All are derived from the Camellia sinensis plant, a shrub native to China and India, and contain unique antioxidants called flavonoids. Tea stimulates stem cells. The more stem cells you have, the longer you will live.

Regarded for thousands of years in the East as a key to good health, tea has caught the attention of researchers in the West, who are discovering the many health benefits of several types of teas. Studies have found that some teas may help with heart disease, cancer, and diabetes. Tea helps with weight loss, lowers cholesterol, and brings about mental alertness.

Although a lot of questions remain unanswered about how long or how much tea needs to be consumed for the most benefit, most experts agree drinking tea is a good thing. I prefer brewed teas over bottled to avoid the extra calories and sweeteners.

What You Need to Know About Different Kinds of Tea

Here is a primer to get you started. It's time to make tea, with its wide varieties, your preferred go-to beverage. Black tea has more caffeine, so it can keep you alert. Have it in the morning. Herbal teas are great for lung health. Peppermint tea helps with indigestion.

Green tea is more than just a hydrating beverage. It is the king of all teas because it contains a range of healthy compounds including catechins or epigallocatechin-3 gallate (EGCG). Catechins are natural antioxidants that help prevent cell damage and provide other benefits.

Research has tested EGCG's ability to help treat various diseases. EGCG has been found in studies to have anticancer effects, reduce inflammation, and help prevent heart and brain disease. Matcha green tea is even more powerful than green tea because it's concentrated. Mix a little unsweetened matcha powder with some almond or coconut milk and ice, and you will have a nice, refreshing drink. White tea is baby green tea, which has even more antioxidants than green tea.

I take you to Turkey now. Winter tea is native to Turkey and has a blend of cinnamon, ginger, turmeric, and pink rose bud. This tea helps fight colds and boost your immune system. It is a good way to get many spices in one drink.

Moving on to China, I love a Chinese tea for its effect on the hallmarks of aging. Jiaogulan tea is native to China, which most people likely have never heard of. People in the original local region of China where jiaogulan, or gynostemma, was traditionally taken were found to have longer lifespans, less disease, and greater vitality than just about any other people in the world. This discovery prompted researchers to study this herb. They discovered that certain plant saponins known as "gypenosides" seem to be responsible for the many benefits of gynostemma. This compound appears to stop the DNA from being degraded and broken down too quickly, and chromosomal instability is one of the ten hallmarks of aging. Gynostemma has been found to stop and even reverse the process of erosion of the telomeres, another hallmark of aging. The effects of gynostemma on telomeres make it one of the most powerful longevity substances ever known.

Recent research indicates that gynostemma actually contains over eighty different saponins compared to the twenty-eight found in ginseng, making it even more powerful. It supports production of nitric oxide, which protects nerve cells from damage and cell death from free radical damage. The saponins in gynostemma exert a regulatory effect on the body. It has positive cardioprotective and immune systems effects. So it's smart to add this drink to your daily routine. You can also take jiaogulan as a supplement.

A Patient's Story

Sharon, a fifty-year-old woman, came to see me because she was concerned about her overall health. She exercised regularly and was not overweight, but she was often fatigued and had high cholesterol and elevated blood pressure. She had frequent feelings of bloating and suffered from chronic diarrhea, and she wanted to know what she might be doing wrong. Her diet was not awful. She ate a lot of fish, chicken, and fruit and avoided processed foods and fast food. After an extensive workup, I diagnosed Sharon with SIBO, or small intestinal bacterial overgrowth, which means bad bacteria taking over the good bacteria in the gut. So I asked Sharon to add some superfoods into her diet. To help with her gut, she added kimchi and kefir, and she started eating a lot more berries and fiber-rich vegetables and replaced some animal protein with beans. She traded her occasional diet soda for tea. After a few months, her stomach issues were gone. Her cholesterol and blood pressure normalized, and she had much more energy—telling me she felt like she did when she was in her twenties.

As you can see, there are many things at your disposal that can target several hallmarks of aging. I try to make great choices every day. I make my lemonade with the whole lemon. I may choose to toss some broccoli or cauliflower on my salads. I frequently drink green tea and jiaogulan tea, and I take them in pill form too. I am truly throwing the kitchen sink at all the hallmarks of aging. I am not restricted to one Blue Zone or one country. My journey to live better has made me experience foods from all over the world.

Remember . . .

- Include lots of superfoods in your diet such as beans, cruciferous vegetables, and seafood.

- Eat vegetables and fruits with various colors.

- Go for wild fish.

- Medium-chain triglycerides such as those found in coconuts are used for energy and not storage.

- Drink a variety of teas. Drink green tea frequently. Matcha green tea powder is also a great choice.

- Explore other exotic tea options like jiaogulan from China.

CHAPTER 11

Spice Up Your Food and Live Longer

Spices are the magic ingredients that make our
food delicious and nutritious.
—**Rachael Ray**

Aging is great if you know how to handle it with knowledge and wisdom. I wish I had known about healthy eating in my twenties. I would have embraced it with enthusiasm. Back then, my kitchen was full of cereals with tons of chemicals. My refrigerator was stocked with various commercially prepared salad dressings made with soybean oil, fat-free yogurt, margarine, and other things I shouldn't have been eating. When I got educated and learned the truth, I completely changed my diet. You can do this too, reverse the cellular damage and improve your longevity. It's never too late to get young.

Back in the 1960s, the microbiologist Leonard Hayflick discovered that human cells divide from forty to sixty times until they reach the Hayflick limit and stop. Eventually, cells can't perform necessary functions like clearing damaged proteins, repairing DNA, and dying. But if we ensure that our cells are as healthy as possible, we can extend their life cycles beyond this limit.

Longevity: The Power of Spices

For millennia, humans have explored ways to achieve agelessness. While no one has found the actual fountain of youth, scientists are rediscovering plant-based remedies that can improve health and longevity.

You've already learned about superfoods, but spices are superstars or even supernovas thanks to the nutrients they contain, how they affect your metabolism, and that they target the ten hallmarks of aging. These humble heroes of your pantry and staples of countries in the Blue Zones can actually affect how your cells perform long term. Longevity is possible if you can unlock the potential of your DNA to slow down the aging process. Adding spices like turmeric, garlic, cinnamon, ginseng, ginger, and za'atar is a great place to start. Let's take a closer look at these spices and how they improve health and longevity.

Turmeric

Turmeric is delicious, with an earthy, bitter pepper-like flavor. It's that deep, insistent flavor you'll find in most curry powders. Turmeric's color is a deep ochre, an orangey-yellow that will stain your table linens and sometimes fingers (and face) if you are not careful. But it is always worth it for its complex flavor.

This superstar nutrient provides anti-aging benefits, because of its anti-inflammatory properties, thanks to curcumin. Chronic inflammation can lead to problems like arthritis, heart disease, and cancer.

Turmeric can speed up recovery after a muscle injury or a workout. A 2017 study in *The FASEB Journal* found that participants in numerous studies who supplemented with curcumin had less overall muscle soreness and faster recovery times than those who did not. How we feel as we age has to do with how our bodies respond to the activities that we once took for granted. Inhibited movement is bad because it can cause depression and make us less likely to be active. Unlike medications that address many of the same problems, turmeric has no side effects and is gentle on your stomach. So it's time to learn how to cook curry dishes, add turmeric to your morning smoothie, or use it in baking (your food will taste great and have a beautiful color). Enjoy Asian dishes like shrimp curry made with turmeric. Have turmeric as a small shot at your local juice store. Try a turmeric latte instead of a sugary Frappuccino. If you take a turmeric pill as a supplement, it is important to take piperine with it as well as it enhances its absorption.

Garlic

Garlic grows all over the world, is produced in different forms, and has been a part of most cultures' culinary histories. Whether garlic is added to a curry dish, a marinara sauce, or a truly authentic boeuf bourguignon, it is everywhere.

This indispensable vegetable is more than just tasty. It has a long history of medicinal qualities such as detoxification, anti-oxidation, antifungal activity, antibacterial activity, tumor suppression, and, you guessed it, anti-aging and rejuvenating effects too. One of its rejuvenating effects is garlic's ability to reverse wrinkles, dark pigmentations, and other effects of aging caused by UV rays, smoking, and stress. The skin's degradation happens because its collagen—the stuff that keeps your skin hydrated, bouncy, and firm—becomes compromised. Garlic can promote the generation of new collagen cells and roll back the years, erasing youthful mistakes like sunbathing or indulging in Marlboro Reds.

Garlic's antioxidant, antifungal, and antibacterial qualities fight off harmful agents that invariably lead to the accumulation of toxins, illness, and disease. Eat garlic raw, in all kinds of foods, or take it as a supplement. If you do not like the garlic smell, roasting it takes away its pungency and gives it a sweet and nutty flavor.

Cinnamon

Cinnamon, the rolled bark of the Southeast Asian tree species *Cinnamomum*, is often used as a seasoning for savory and sweet foods. There are two types: cinnamon cassia, which is quite common and may already be in your pantry, and Ceylon cinnamon.

Ceylon cinnamon, with its lighter color and delicate taste, is much safer and has anti-inflammatory properties like garlic and turmeric. Cinnamon can also inhibit the breakdown of collagen, regenerate it, and give skin a youthful look.

Cinnamon can help balance your immune system, is antiparasitic, can alleviate the symptoms of autoimmune diseases like multiple sclerosis, promotes gut health, helps manage colitis, and can even protect the brain. It has been shown that cinnamon reduces the risk of Alzheimer's disease by preventing one of the main characteristics of the disease, tau protein, from forming.

Happily, cinnamon is one of the most loved spices in many cultures and takes a star turn in baked goods, adds fragrance to stews and tagines, and can dust the top of your cappuccino. No matter how you choose to incorporate it into your diet, cinnamon is a workhorse that should be placed front and center in your pantry.

Research shows that Ceylon cinnamon can help reduce blood pressure and support a healthy heart. It helps brain function and may halt Alzheimer's disease. To get the maximum benefits of cinnamon, I take it in pill form.

Ginger

Ginger not only makes your food taste great and your home smell good but it is also another pantry hero for its anti-inflammatory and antioxidant properties, key to health and longevity. Ginger, which can be consumed in its dried and powdered form, fresh as an extract, or even pickled, not only helps you live longer but makes you *want* to live longer by impacting cellular health and reducing inflammation.

Ginger is well-known for its ability to combat nausea that is brought on by chemotherapy, pregnancy, motion sickness, and so many other illnesses. Ginger can also help you treat indigestion naturally rather than relying on over-the-counter medications taken for heartburn, acid reflux, gas, and other effects of overeating or eating the wrong foods.

Ginger also inhibits brain inflammation, which causes cognitive deterioration, and may help lower your LDL cholesterol and reduce common menstrual pain. Applied either as a topical cream or ingested orally, it can also reduce the pain and stiffness brought on by osteoarthritis.

Both ginger and turmeric are rhizomes (roots) from the same genus and can be used in the same dishes. I love ginger chicken and enjoy having a ginger shot whenever I go to the juice store.

Ginseng

Ginseng refers to eleven different varieties for a slow-growing plant with fleshy roots. It can help lower sugar levels, lower cholesterol, promote relaxation, and improve sexual dysfunction in men, and is used to treat a wide range of medical conditions. It helps with cognitive function and flu prevention. Researchers believe that ginsenosides are responsible for the clinical effects of the herb. Take it daily as a supplement or add it to your dishes or juice. A word of caution: taking more than two grams a day can increase the risk of bleeding.

Cardamom

Cardamom, or cardamon, is a spice made from the seeds of several plants found in India and Indonesia with a unique taste. There are two types, green and black. Green cardamom is used mostly in Asian cuisines, and black cardamom adds a dash of smoky flavor in your meals.

Cardamom has antioxidant, anti-inflammatory, and skin anti-aging properties and may help lower blood pressure. Cardamom has compounds that enhance natural killer cells to attack cancer cells. A word of caution: if you are pregnant, be careful—there are reports of miscarriage with excess use of cardamom.

Saffron

Saffron is a brightly colored spice that is high in health-promoting compounds. It can be used for cooking or taken as a supplement. Derived from the Crocus sativus flower, saffron is harvested by hand, which contributes to high production costs and makes it the most expensive spice in the world. Saffron probably originated in Persia (current-day Iran), and while Saffron's origin is debated, its medicinal properties are not. Saffron is a powerful anti-oxidant. It helps with mood and depressive symptoms.

In a review of five studies, saffron supplements were more effective than placebos at treating mild to moderate depression symptoms. At 30 mg, it was as effective as the antidepressant fluoxetine. Saffron also has anticancer properties. The benefits of this wonderful spice don't stop here. Saffron helps reduce PMS symptoms, acts as an aphrodisiac, helps to reduce appetite, and may assist with weight loss. Saffron also helps lower blood sugar as well as help to reduce heart disease risk and assists to improve memory in Alzheimer's disease patients.

It is important to note that when you buy saffron, it should be from a reputable source. The product should come in a closed tin, not a plastic bag exposed to the light. You can also take saffron as a supplement at a dose of 30 mg a day.

Za'atar

We go to the Middle East again to learn about za'atar. Za'atar is a blend of various spices with antioxidant and anti-aging properties. The ratios change, but it is usually a mix of dried oregano and/or thyme, sesame seeds, and sumac. Sometimes, cumin, coriander, and anise are used as well. In some parts of the Middle East, the mix is brightened with lemon zest. The great Spanish Jewish philosopher Maimonides gave it to his patients in the twelfth century to improve their health and treat a wide range of illnesses. Rub on your meat before cooking for the various benefits.

As you can see, a Western diet lacks the nutrition found in those spices. Although most of us don't live in the Blue Zones, we can still benefit from these superfoods, and spices each day. For example, I have vegetable juice with some ginger, ginseng, and turmeric once or twice a week. It is a fast way to add super nutrients to my diet without going crazy looking for these exotic foods. I also have some za'atar and turmeric in my kitchen to use as a rub on poultry and to cook simple dishes. When eating out, I go for salads made with avocados, nuts, mushrooms, and berries instead of croutons and bacon bits. I also take Ceylon cinnamon in pill form. It's easy to incorporate all the superfoods into my diet. Again, targeting the hallmarks of aging should be a no-brainer when you have the knowledge.

You can do the same. You'll feel good knowing that you're doing all you can to be healthy and improve your longevity. Later in this book, you'll find a collection of recipes that have all been designed to nourish you with these spices.

Remember . . .

- Make sure to include many spices in your diet such as turmeric, saffron, and ginger.
- Go for Ceylon cinnamon. It is better for your health.
- Take spices as supplements, such as a turmeric or saffron pill daily if you do not like the taste of those spices.
- Always follow a balanced diet with a variety of spices.

CHAPTER 12

Eat Clean and Live Longer

Take care of your body.
It's the only place you have to live.
—Jim Rohn

It is a dirty little secret that no one wants to acknowledge: much of our hormonal imbalance comes from the environmental assault on us from toxins and pesticides. Low testosterone in men and irregular periods in women are perfect examples. Pesticides have been linked to Parkinson's disease in some people, and even some forms of cancer. Toxins and pesticides damage our DNA. It is no wonder organic foods rule. According to a new study in the journal *Environmental Research,* people who switched from a conventional to an organic diet reduced their intake of pesticides by 60 percent in just one week! But who can afford organic food with all its extra costs?

For this reason, this chapter is dedicated to showing you that *The Ageless Revolution* is financially feasible—you simply need to make the right choices. Choosing less expensive protein sources such as mushrooms and beans, and organic chicken rather than red meat can help you stretch your budget so you can buy more organic vegetables.

Affordable Protein Choices on *The Ageless Revolution*

Beans

Cottage cheese

Eggs

Greek yogurt

Mushrooms

Poultry

Remember protein should be 10 to 15 percent of your calories. You can go to 20 percent if you work out, do anaerobic activity, and are over thirty. Seafood is also a great protein choice, but it is costly.

Our Toxic World

We are living in a toxic world. We eat chemicals. We ingest pesticides. Toxins enter our bodies through the skin, the food, and the air we breathe. The longer you are on this earth, the more likely you are going to have toxins in your body. You have about 37 trillion cells in your body, and if you do not take the toxins out, the cells will be impaired. Toxins impair your DNA. Chromosomal instability is one of the ten hallmarks of aging. So it's time to take toxicity seriously.

What You'll Learn About Eating Clean

In this chapter, you'll learn about the dangers of pesticide-contaminated produce, and the sometimes misleading language on all food labels, so you can be certain you are making healthy choices as you embark on this new journey.

Here is the dirt on eating clean: pesticides, including insecticides, herbicides, and fungicides, are harmful to your well-being and the planet's future. Your body responds to all the unseen elements inside the foods you eat, whether they are beneficial or poisonous.

The Dangers of Pesticides

Pesticides are killing agents used in farming to reduce crop damage and increase the harvest of fruits, vegetables, and other crops. Food stores also use a variety of pesticides to keep pests away from their stockrooms. We often use them in our homes and gardens too.

Pesticides are used to kill weeds, rodents, insects, molds, fungus, and anything else that stands in the way of a good harvest, a lovely golf course, a pretty patio, or a picture-perfect fruit or vegetable.

Soil holds bacteria, nematodes, fungi, and many other microbes. Some might be considered harmful, but most are beneficial and essential for healthy soil and plants. The natural variety of insects, amphibians, and birds decreases with pesticide use too. Just think about the declining bee population.

Just as the overuse of antibiotics can cause some germs to become resistant, the overuse of pesticides can create superweeds. Some insects and pathogens can become resistant to pesticides, so what happens? More powerful and different pesticides are manufactured. And we consume all that!

Pesticides are nasty and seep from the soil into the foods we eat, contributing to many health problems, including nervous system damage, hormonal imbalance in both men and women, and neurologic and developmental illnesses in children. They can lead to the development of Parkinson's disease and have been linked to certain types of cancer like non-Hodgkin's lymphoma. Endangering our health is too high a price to pay for cheaper, bigger, but not better crops. The higher cost of buying organic produce is small by comparison.

Why Organic Food Is Better for Your Health and Longevity

Organic produce, especially strawberries, has more vitamin C and antioxidants than nonorganic strawberries. And they taste better too. In Europe, many of the dangerous pesticides used in the United States are totally banned.

Of course, nonorganic farmers and lobbyists often insist that organically and conventionally produced foods have the same nutrients. But it's difficult to believe that pesticides that kill insects, rodents, molds, and fungus have no adverse effect on the nutritional value of the fruit or vegetable itself or on us.

The Pesticide Action Network (PAN) explains that "chemicals can trigger cancer in a variety of ways, including disrupting hormones, damaging DNA, inflaming tissues and turning genes on and off. Many pesticides are known or probable carcinogens and exposure to these chemicals is widespread." Both the FDA and EPA say that the pesticide residue on produce is still within "safe" limits. But how safe can consuming one to almost two pounds of pesticides a year be? In one study by the Environmental Working Group (EWG), about 70 percent of nonorganic food had residue of one or more harmful chemicals.

Some citrus fruit samples tested positive for the residues of the pesticide imazalil. The suspected carcinogen was even detected on contaminated flesh of peeled oranges. Imazalil, also known as enilconazole, may cause leukocytosis (a too high white blood cell count) and accumulate in various organs. It is also a potential endocrine disruptor and can harm the immune system.

Atrazine, a weed killer, was banned in the European Union in 2004 but is still used in the United States! It is an endocrine disruptor that is especially harmful to women because it can cause menstrual irregularities, low estrogen, fertility issues, and can lead to birth defects. Unbalanced hormones and toxins totally impair cellular communications, a hallmark of aging.

In nature, atrazine can cause male frogs to become sterile, and even unable to mate, which has adversely affected the frog population in some areas.

Organophosphates, specifically chlorpyrifos, have caused convulsions, coma, and death to farmers who had extended, high exposure. The residue was also found in the farmers' homes, where children were exposed and harmed too. Chronic exposure to this dangerous compound attacks the brain and nervous system of insects and mammals and causes infertility in women and low sperm count in men. The origin of this pesticide is horrifying: the Nazis developed it to use in chemical warfare!

Used in the United States since 1966, even low exposure to chlorpyrifos was linked to learning disabilities, neurological problems, and developmental delays in children. Who knows the extent of such damage over fifty-plus years!

Glyphosate is the active ingredient in the weed killer Roundup. There have been many lawsuits filed because it has been linked to an increased risk of non-Hodgkin's lymphoma. However, the EPA says glyphosate is unlikely to be a carcinogen, based on unpublished research studies provided by Monsanto—the manufacturer of Roundup.

Recently, the EPA approved a new pesticide, Enlist Duo, which combines 2,4-D with glyphosate. Studies show that 2,4-D may be an endocrine disruptor. It was once an ingredient in Agent Orange, the toxic defoliant used in the Vietnam War. Neonicotinoids, commonly referred to as neonics, are suspected to have decimated bee colonies. As an insecticide, neonics accumulate in the soil and also kill nontargeted insects like earthworms, an invertebrate.

Paraquat is a weed killer that has been linked to the development of Parkinson's disease even when inhaled at low exposure. It is banned in China and the European Union, but not in the United States!

I don't mean to beat around the bush here, but I think you get the picture. In the Blue Zones, they eat what is in their backyards, the wild vegetables and fruits provide them with daily super nutrients. Their food also tastes better since it's natural and contains zero chemicals.

Best Practices when Eating Fruits and Vegetables

Whether you go organic or non-organic, always wash your fruits and vegetables carefully. First, wash your hands with soap and water. Clean the utensils, sinks, and surfaces you are using too. Use cool water for the produce. Do not use soap or commercial cleaners: they are unnecessary and harmful.

Fruits with an outer covering—like citrus fruits, bananas, and pineapples—are less prone to pesticide contamination. But rinse them well anyway before peeling. Then rewash your hands so you do not carry any residue from the outer skin to the inner flesh. Cut away any very bruised or visibly rotted areas of fresh fruit. Firm produce like apples, lemons, and pears and root vegetables like potatoes, carrots, and turnips can be cleaned with a soft brush to remove residue from their pores.

Remove and throw away the outer leaves of greens like spinach, lettuce, and kale. Brussels sprouts and broccoli have more dirt-trapping layers. Soak them in cool water, then rinse and drain them. If you need to, pat them dry with a clean kitchen towel. Go to your local farmers' market on weekends and save money. Local farmers' markets are cheaper than big organic supermarket chains.

The Dirty Dozen

Below you will find a list of vegetables and fruits that are prone to having high levels of pesticides. They are called the dirty dozen. You should try to buy them organic. This list is updated each year by the Environmental Working Group (EWG).

Strawberries

Grapes

Apples

Spinach

Nectarine

Pears

Peaches

Cherries

Green beans

Blueberries

Kale, collard, mustard greens

Bell and hot peppers

Labels Aren't Perfect

The United States Department of Agriculture (USDA) does its best to give us an idea of what we are eating. Not all labeling is perfect, but you will be better informed if you know what the labels mean. The term *GMO* stands for genetically modified organisms (plant, microbe), but it is being replaced by "bioengineered food."

Bottom line? Most of the food we eat today has been altered in one shape or another. Companies are required to disclose whether their products contain GMOs, but they do not have to make it easy for consumers. Instead of using the "bioengineered" label, companies can include a QR code, web address, or phone number so consumers have to do their own research. Most don't.

Keep in mind that to date, there is no scientific consensus about the safety of GMO foods, and the approval process for new GMO products is conducted by the same companies that sell those products. So, it's safer to avoid it. Buy fruits and vegetables at a local farmer's market or go to the organic section of your local supermarket.

Meats and Poultry

More bad news: our animal food supply is not safe either. Today, most animals are given hormones, which are passed on to us and negatively affect the IGF-1, a nutrient-sensing pathway. High levels of the IGF-1 pathway have been linked to increased mortality in elderly women.

Nonorganic red meat is also high in omega-6 fatty acids that cause inflammation. Grass-fed cows (as they should be, not grain-fed) contain omega-3 fatty acids, which fight inflammation. Whoever thought to give cows corn and grains to eat? Cows love bread. All USDA-inspected meat and poultry must have a USDA seal of inspection and a code for the producing establishment. Meat and egg labels with a grade (like USDA Grade A beef or jumbo eggs) are based on quality and size, not production methods. Private certification programs vary in their standards.

A Deeper Dive into Labels

No Antibiotics Administered or *Raised Without Antibiotics* means the animal was not given any antibiotic during its entire life. However, large facilities often feed the animals low doses of antibiotics to prevent disease developing in their often-crammed facilities. This process kills our gut flora at the same time, which we need for longevity.

Raised Without Added Hormones, No Synthetic Hormones, No Hormones Administered means, as they say, that no hormones were given to the animal; however, it says nothing about their feed, living conditions, or if they were given antibiotics. Eating hormone-treated meat is believed to cause human health problems that include a risk of cancer and early-onset puberty.

Often, hormones are given to dairy cows to regulate their cycles so they can be artificially inseminated more often, give birth, and increase milk production. This nonorganic milk is full of hormones that are bad for us. Male calves are immediately slaughtered because they do not produce milk. Dairy, in excess, is linked to prostate cancer in men. So choose plant-based milks such as coconut or almond milk instead on *The Ageless Revolution.*

Free-Range might only mean the chickens have been outside for a brief time and not necessarily every day. The USDA approves this label only for chickens raised for meat, not egg-laying chickens. Likewise, *Cage-Free* can overlook that chickens raised for eggs could be indoors in overcrowded factory farms. *Grass-Fed* means that after weaning, the animal ate grass or forage of unknown quality. It does not exclude the use of antibiotics or hormones. *Pasture-Raised* means the animals spent at least some of their lives outdoors, feeding on grass and forage. There is no metric for how much time. A label that says *Fresh* can also be misleading or inadequate. This just means that poultry was not cooled below 26°F. It must be labeled frozen if it reaches zero degrees. The label does not mean that any type of meat has not been processed or preserved in some way. The USDA does not define or regulate the use of the *Fresh* label on any other type of product.

According to the USDA, *Natural* and *Naturally Raised* means that the meat and poultry cannot contain artificial colors, flavors, or preservatives, and should be "minimally" processed. Again, it says nothing about how animals were raised, fed, or if antibiotics and hormones were used.

With so many misleading labels, it's easy to become confused about which toxins we're consuming. The best rule of thumb is to eat natural, organic foods. While it's not practical to buy our own farms to stay alive, we can make better choices. Go to your local farmers' markets on weekends. Buy foraged food online. Eat more beans, wild fish, organic vegetables, and fruits, especially the ones that are on the dangerous list. When you do your best to eat clean, you can, in fact, change your DNA, genetic destiny, health, and longevity.

Remember . . .

- *Pesticide exposure or ingestion* is harmful, even deadly. It damages your DNA. Use natural fertilizers and pest control in your garden and stay away from large areas that you see being commercially landscaped or gardened as dangerous pesticides were probably used.

- *Wash produce,* especially nonorganic produce. Wash your hands, utensils, sink, surfaces, and then produce. Use cool water. Rinse all fruits and vegetables. Peel fruit with thick skin such as bananas, mangoes, then wash your hands again. Cut away bruised or rotting parts and use a soft brush on firm produce like carrots. Throw away the outer leaves of greens like lettuce, then soak the rest in water, rinse, and pat dry.

- Learn to read labels. It is so important for your longevity.

- *No Antibiotics* means the animal has never, in its entire life, received antibiotic treatment.

- *Raised Without Hormones* might be true, but it says nothing about the feed, antibiotics, or the conditions where the animal was raised and later held.

- *USDA inspected* means the meat and poultry are of good grade, quality, and size. It says nothing about production methods that can include GMOs, antibiotics, or hormones.

- *Pasture-Raised* and *Free-Range* mean some nonspecific portion of animal's life was spent outdoors. This does not apply to egg-laying chickens.

- *Cage-Free* is the term used but they could be in crowded, hangar-like, indoor facilities.

- The USDA label *Fresh* will appear only on poultry. It means the product has not been cooled under 26 degrees and has never been frozen.

- *Natural* or *Naturally Raised* indicates that the product was minimally processed with no artificial colors, flavors, or preservatives added.

- *The Bottom Line:* Whenever you can, go to your local farmers' market and choose organic fruits and vegetables. Eat fewer animal products.

- *Eat wild food more often.* You can buy wild food from online websites.

CHAPTER 13

Gut Health and Longevity

All disease begins in the gut.
—Hippocrates

Gut health is so important for longevity that I've named it the tenth hallmark of aging. Fermented foods like kimchi, sauerkraut, yogurt, cheese, miso, natto (fermented soybeans), and kefir contain helpful bacteria that improve gut health and are eaten frequently in the Blue Zones. A healthy gut means healthy aging and improved longevity. So this means we must make healthy gut flora a top priority and an ally in our health.

What You Need to Know About Gut Flora

Forty trillion flora or bacteria live in our gut. Humans have evolved to live with these microbes for millions of years. Yes, these bacteria help to digest fiber, but they do so much more. Healthy gut flora can improve immune function, heart health, brain health, and weight.

When people say they have a gut feeling something is right or wrong, or they have butterflies in their stomach, they are not wrong. Your gut is your second brain, and gut bacteria affect emotions. Serotonin, a neurotransmitter that improves mood, is mainly created in the gut. We have both beneficial bacteria and bad bacteria in our gut. So it's important to keep both in balance to have a healthy gut environment. To have beneficial bacteria in our gut, we need prebiotics and probiotics in our diet. Each plays an important role in your health.

Prebiotics are the fiber found in vegetables and fruits that gut bacteria feed upon. Without prebiotics, healthy bacteria can't fight off unhealthy bacteria in the gut as effectively. Prebiotics support digestive health, support the immune system, promote healthy inflammatory response, help support healthy cholesterol levels, and boost a healthy metabolism. Because they supply bulk that makes you feel full, prebiotics can also support weight loss.

Probiotics are live bacteria you will find in some fermented foods such as sauerkraut, kimchi, yogurt, kefir, and supplements. These bacteria help control your metabolism, make vitamin K and other essential chemicals, affect how medicines work, boost your immune system and heart health, lower cancer risk, protect the layers of your large intestine with fatty acids, and keep inflammation at bay. All these functions are important to reach your ageless goals.

Overuse of Antibiotics Impacts Our Gut Bacteria

The excess use of antibiotics can be detrimental to our longevity. Antibiotics help when it comes to treating a bacterial illness but can also impact gut bacteria negatively. That's because antibiotics kill beneficial bacteria along with the bad, leaving you with a poor defense against illness. And once your gut bacteria are wiped out, it can take up to two years to replenish them!

Probiotics are necessary to offset the harm of antibiotics. Many of my patients insist that I give them an antibiotic when they come down with any infection, even a viral one. I explain to them that this won't help but will wipe out beneficial gut bacteria.

You can also consume antibiotics from the nonorganic animal products you eat. Often animals are injected with antibiotics to keep them from getting sick as they are being fattened up for slaughter. They may also be given hormones to make them bigger and grow faster, and other substances that are unhealthy for humans. This impairs the IGF-1 pathway, the nutrient-sensing pathway in your cells. This is a particularly good reason to buy only organic produce, eggs, milk, wild salmon, organic chicken, and meat from grass-fed cows.

Good Dental Hygiene and Bad Bacteria

To get a handle on your gut bacteria, it should start in your mouth. You can control the type and number of bacteria that enter your body, and your toothbrush is the first line of defense. The wrong bacteria can eat away the enamel of your teeth. To keep those invaders at bay, brush and floss your teeth at least twice a day and clean your tongue too. Not only will you prevent tooth decay and gum disease, but you will rid your mouth of bad bacteria as well.

Poor oral hygiene can cause *system-wide* inflammation. Inflammation, as you know, is the root of age-related diseases including Alzheimer's and cardiovascular disease. Poor gum and teeth health have been linked to endocarditis, or inflammation of the inner lining of the heart.

Gut Health in the Blue Zones

A surprising number of people living in those areas live a hundred years or longer. Part of the reason is that each meal includes fiber-rich foods like whole grains, nuts, vegetables, beans, and fresh fruit that promote healthy gut bacteria. Fiber helps feed your gut bacteria so that you can keep a diverse and healthy balance. Prebiotics are found in many vegetables, fruits, and legumes including berries, Jerusalem artichokes, asparagus, dandelion greens, leeks, and onions.

Probiotics are also popular in the Blue Zones and can be found in fermented foods like sauerkraut, organic yogurt, cottage cheese, traditional (not cultured) buttermilk, kamancheh, tempeh, whole milk kefir, and fermented foods. Ikaria favors yogurt. Sardinia prefers sheep's cheese. In Okinawa, tofu and miso paste are the top choices.

Gut Bacteria, Cellular Health, and Longevity

Gut bacteria help us live longer by protecting the mitochondria. As you've learned, mitochondrial dysfunction is one of the ten hallmarks of aging. You need the battery of your cells to be fully charged and optimized.

Polyphenolic compounds such as urolithin A (UA) and ellagic acid (EA), and ellagitannins (ET) such as punicalagin are produced by gut bacteria when we eat certain foods. These are dietary polyphenolic compounds that include ellagic acid (EA) and ellagitannins (ET, which are found widely in fruits (pomegranate and certain berries) and nuts (walnuts and pecans). ET is converted to EA in the upper part of the human gastrointestinal tract, and further metabolized by gut microflora in the large intestine into compounds known as urolithins, of which UA is among the most common. Urolithin (UA) protects mitochondria—the battery of our cells, which is imperative for our overall health. It is important to note that individuals show significant differences in urolithin production capacity due to variations in the microbiome responsible for ET metabolism. So it may be wise to add urolithin as a supplement for many of us. In summary or simple terms, certain fruits with the help of gut bacteria make compounds like urolithin, which protects the mitochondria. But that's not the only reason gut health is so important for our health.

Gut bacteria also make vitamin K2, which prevents heart disease. Heart disease is the number one killer in the Western world for both men and women. Vitamin K2 prevents calcium from being deposited in the arteries. Gut bacteria also play a role in our weight. They help us with our metabolism. Now we can understand the immense role of gut health in longevity.

Sugar Has a Negative Effective on Gut Bacteria

Sugar is not only bad for your waistline but bad for your gut bacteria too. If you regularly feed the wrong bacteria with sugar, they grow faster and colonize more easily. This means that there are less good bacteria to keep the bad ones in check.

Cut out sugar, low-fat products, and artificial sweeteners from your diet. Limit processed supermarket honey too. Manuka honey and monk fruit are great alternatives for your sweet tooth. They are easy to find at your local grocery store.

Prebiotic and Probiotic Supplements

Hate fermented products? Dislike yogurt? Want to take a probiotic supplement instead as a shortcut to gut health? I am afraid this is not the answer. I do not recommend this easy route to gut health. There are many prebiotics (fiber) and probiotic supplements on the market. You might prefer a daily pill, capsule, powder, or liquid supplement.

Unless you do your research, you may be wasting your money. Live bacteria may not be consistent in the varied brands, or even within the same brand's manufacturer. Some probiotic supplements are not effective because they don't survive stomach acid and make it to your large intestine. So you need to determine what strain you need, exactly what's in the product formula, and how to store it. People who are suffering from small intestine bacterial overgrowth (SIBO) have too many probiotics in their systems already, so they should not take a probiotic supplement. It can make their symptoms worse.

The first step in the longevity path is to change your diet, so it's best to get your prebiotics and probiotics from real food. If you have any stomach or gut issues you should consult with a health-care professional who is knowledgeable about gut health.

I can't emphasize enough how little measures that you can implement can make a huge difference in your life. It is easy to look after your gut bacteria like the folks in the Blue Zones. At Korean restaurants, try kimchi. Have some full-fat yogurt or kefir in your refrigerator. They make great breakfast or fast snacks. Cut sugar from your diet. All these little things long term will add up to have a huge impact.

Remember . . .

- Your gut health is important for longevity as your gut bacteria make compounds that protect the mitochondria.

- Gut bacteria also affect your brain health as they affect the nervous system.

- *Prebiotics* are the fiber that provides food for gut bacteria. Eat green vegetables, fruit, legumes, berries, Jerusalem artichokes, asparagus, dandelion greens, leeks, and onions.

- *Probiotics* are fermented products. This good bacteria helps control metabolism, make vitamin K and other essential chemicals, make medications work, and boost the immune system and heart health. Eat yogurt, kefir, traditional buttermilk, kimchi, kombucha, tempeh, and other fermented foods.

- *Mitochondria* are the batteries of your cells. Gut health is essential to support their health.

- *Another reason to eliminate sugar*: it feeds the bad bacteria, helping them grow and overtake the healthy bacteria.

- Take *antibiotics* only when you need them but remember that too much too often will destroy good bacteria along with the bad.

- *Brush your teeth* at least twice a day and scrape your tongue too. Bad bacteria in your mouth can cause serious systemic inflammation.

PART IV

The Ageless Revolution

CHAPTER 14

Becoming Ageless with Intermittent Fasting

Coming out of your comfort zone is tough in the beginning, chaotic in the middle, and awesome in the end.
—**Manoj Arora**

So far, you've learned how lifestyle, diet, and maintaining healthy gut flora are the fundamental first steps to change your genetic destiny. As I've shown you, epigenetic alteration affects the interpretation of your DNA. Think of epigenetic alteration like a conductor of a symphony, and the musicians are the genes. Your life is the music that comes out of it. The conductor may silence some musicians, or he can make some musicians up their game. The end result is vastly different if the conductor never conducted a symphony before or he was from the New York Philharmonic. You are in control. You are the conductor. So, congratulations for having come this far! You're learning about new, effective ways to move forward and reverse your biological age. It is time to make some great music. Next on your to-do list is intermittent fasting. Why? Because intermittent fasting activates sirtuins.

What Is Intermittent Fasting?

So what is intermittent fasting? It is based on short periods of not eating—no more than sixteen hours—or eating at certain times of the day. The goal of fasting is to avoid age-related diseases. Fasting alerts your hero proteins, sirtuins, yelling, "We are here to help!" as they recognize you are experiencing the physical stress of hunger or starvation. They charge in to kick up gene activity to levels that will keep you alive. And those sirtuins stimulate the protein complex mTOR that builds cells after a process called autophagy, which clears out (eats) dead and dying cells, which improves longevity.

Most health experts tell us to eat every three hours. People with cancer are told to eat a proper diet while undergoing chemotherapy. Work by Valter Longo, an Italian American biogerontologist, shows that the exact opposite is true. In fact, Longo recommends intermittent fasting even for cancer patients undergoing chemotherapy. It renders those folks more responsive to chemotherapy. This flies in the face of conventional wisdom that tells cancer patients to eat as much as they can during treatments or what the American Cancer Society recommends. According to the American Cancer Society website, eating well during treatments is essential. I found this on their website: "People with cancer during treatment should snack throughout the day. Have cereal, cheese and crackers, cookies, granola, microwave snacks, muffins, popcorn, pretzels, ice cream, frozen yogurt, and sports drinks!" But research shows cancer starves when there is no sugar. Cancer cells are hungry for sugar. We need to kill the cancer cells, not feed them.

How Practicing Intermittent Fasting Helps the Body

When you skip a meal, the body is alerted that there may be a shortage of food and of a danger ahead. Your life needs to be preserved. So insulin levels and hunger hormones go down. Human growth hormone (HGH), a hormone that preserves muscles, goes up. Your body starts to tap its fat reserves and gets rid of dead protein in cells, other damaged cell parts, and old cells. Amazing.

Like everything you put into or do to your body, intermittent fasting (IF) affects your hormone production. Many things happen in your body on both the molecular and cellular levels.

The effects of practicing IF:

- Your hormone levels change to make stored body fat more accessible and easier to burn off.

- Your cells perform all kinds of repairs throughout your body and change the expression of your genes.

- Your *natural* levels of human growth hormone (HGH) increase severalfold. That makes it easier for your body to get rid of fat and gain lean muscle mass. Increased muscle mass means increased metabolic rates, so that you will burn calories more easily when you are at rest.

- Your insulin levels drop. Once your insulin levels are lowered, it is easier for your body to burn stored fat.

- Your body starts a process called autophagy. That means your cells start repairing themselves by eating and digesting old, misfolded, broken, and no longer useful proteins. It will get rid of the other parts of damaged cells. This new hallmark of aging was added in 2022. The body will also get rid of senescent, or zombie, cells. With that debris out of the way, your cells can now rebuild themselves properly from the inside out. New cells are formed.

- Any cancer cells that are present start to die as the body starts to find alternative sources of energy.

- DNA is triggered to make all sorts of things happen in our bodies, both good and bad. Fasting turns on sirtuins, which is a positive switch that activates longevity.

- IF stimulates the production of a fat-burning hormone called norepinephrine, also known as noradrenaline.

- Hormonal changes help increase muscle mass. Also, it can radically improve the efficacy and speed of your metabolism by 3.6 to 14 percent.

- Ghrelin, the hunger hormone, is suppressed for a few weeks after an extended fast, so you will not be hungry after stopping this extended fast.

You may be saying, "Hey Doc, all this work to find organic food, wild food, fermented products, and eat clean, and now you are telling me to starve my-self?" I am only sharing medical information and the latest research. Nothing in this book is my personal opinion, so please do not shoot the messenger. If you want longevity and a new way to age, it is in your hands. Intermittent fasting can target a few hallmarks of aging as you will soon see.

The first thing to explain is that fasting is nothing new to the human experience. Evolution and natural selection have relentlessly optimized our genes, favoring the strong ones, or survival for the fittest. Evolution does not care if you live long. The evolutionary process did not design for us to eat every three hours. Humans were designed to survive when food is scarce. We were not designed to eat sugar. Over the centuries, fasting has become more sophisticated, so it must be done in between a clean eating plan. Believe me, you will not die if you skip a meal or two in a week.

Here is an example of *extreme* fasting. In 1971, an obese Scottish man by the name of Angus Barbieri was fed up with his morbid weight. He was twenty-seven years old and weighed over 456 pounds. He fasted for 382 days with no food, just water, setting a record! He got down to 180 pounds and set a Guinness World Record for the longest duration of human fasting. This man had tons of fat reserves, so please do not challenge his record. It is just an example to show you how long a human can go without food. You can benefit from fasting too—but in a more sensible way. You will be surprised by all that fasting can do for you.

Before you start thinking I am telling you to starve yourself for an extended period like the Scotsman who reportedly lived on water for 382 days, I am not! Intermittent fasting is based on short periods of not eating—no more than sixteen hours. It is a hard medicine to swallow when we are accustomed to having food around us. My beautiful Yorkie dog cannot stop eating.

He looks at me with his angel eyes, and always wants to eat. When I finally give in an hour later, he vomits everything. He does not know when to stop. Now, I know better. I ignore him as I love him, and I want him to live for a long time. We are no different. We can eat tons of ice cream or other sweets, and we do not know when to stop, or how this excess food is so bad for us. It is so bad for our nutrient-sensing pathways.

How Fasting Affects the Body

Fasting is nothing new to humans. We don't actually need to eat three meals a day or five to six small meals, a plan favored by bodybuilders. This is not how humans were designed. Adversity was the norm in early human life. We went against nature. Frequent eating turns off sirtuins, the repair proteins in your cells. Once collagen or bound sugar molecules in the muscles are used, your body turns into fat. Ketone bodies are produced and used for energy instead of sugar. Researchers found that your system switches to ketone bodies you go into ketosis. Again, this means when your body uses protein and fat as a source of energy instead of sugar. Ketosis indicates elevated levels of ketones, including acetoacetate, beta-hydroxybutyrate (BHB), and acetone, which are water-soluble molecules produced by fatty acids. Ketones are a very efficient source of energy, so fasting is a wonderful way to lose weight, improve insulin, fight off depression, and boost brain functions. Most importantly, natural human growth hormone (HGH) increases, which is important for muscle growth, energy, and longevity when it is secreted naturally.

I am not suggesting prolonged periods of no food, but what happens if you go without food for a few hours, days, or weeks? When you skip meals, your body adjusts. Say you skip lunch one day because you are too busy; you will be hungry at 1 or 2 PM, but by 4 PM, your craving for food will simply vanish.

This is because when there is an extended period between meals, your body starts to secrete high pulses of human growth hormone (HGH), which preserves muscles. Your insulin level goes down too. A few hours later, ghrelin, the appetite hormone, which is produced in your gut, increases and triggers hunger pangs. Ghrelin stays in circulation for two to three hours and then decreases. You were able to skip a meal successfully. You survived intermittent fasting.

Let's say you decided to go for a longer fast; hunger will return. After seventy-two hours, your hunger pain disappears, and you get a sudden burst of energy as your body totally switches from sugar to ketones for its energy needs. At the same time, the brain-derived neurotrophic factor (BDNF) is secreted, a protein produced in nerve cells that helps the brain cells function and grow. BDNF also encourages the increase of new neurons, strengthens them, and improves their communications. For decades, doctors thought brain cells could not regenerate, but this turned out to be not true. BDNF helps regenerate brain cells and can improve Alzheimer's disease.

Bottom line: Fasting can make your brain work better. It can also have positive effects on metabolism. It is a healthier way to lose weight than standard calorie restriction because it also decreases insulin levels and boosts levels of human growth hormone (HGH) and norepinephrine.

Fasting does *not slow* down metabolism or decrease muscle mass as long as you remain active. But it does encourage your body to get rid of bad proteins in your cells, which can speed aging. Remember, loss of stable synthesis of protein is one of the ten hallmarks of aging. This is when the protein made in your cells is not of good quality. Next, your body starts to eat other dead cells, fat cells, and cancer cells.

Some researchers believe that intermittent fasting may be more effective for maintaining lean muscle mass during weight loss than non-fasting diets. You are just not likely to *build* muscle during those fasting periods. Remember that exercising, whether fasting or not, is always important to your health and longevity. A word of caution: make sure to eat enough protein for your body type if you decide to try intermittent fasting. You need to lose fat, not muscles.

History of Intermittent Fasting

Long before Jennifer Aniston, Jennifer Lopez, and Heidi Klum made intermittent fasting popular, the concept existed for hundreds of years. It was documented in the sixteenth century by a businessman named Luigi Cornaro, also known as Alvise Cornaro (1464– or 1467–1566). He was a Venetian nobleman and patron of arts. He is remembered for his books about living long and well. Cornaro even sat for *Tintoretto* for his portrait, which is now displayed in the Galleria Palatina in Florence. When Cornaro was forty, he found himself exhausted and in poor health. He attributed this to a hedonistic lifestyle of excessive eating, drinking, and sexual licentiousness. On the advice of his doctors, he began to adhere to a calorie restricted diet and wrote four books, including *Discourses on the Temperate Life,* which exclaimed the virtues of eating less to live longer. He remained in vigorous health into old age. He died in Padua at the age of 98. In 1911, American writer Upton Sinclair described the benefits of fasting and how it can fight off disease. Next the benefits of fasting were described by the Soviets in the 1970s. Animal research studies followed.

Intermittent Fasting and Ketosis

Researchers found that when your system switches to ketone bodies you go into ketosis. Ketosis indicates elevated levels of ketones, including acetoacetate, beta-hydroxybutyrate (BHB), and acetone, which are water-soluble molecules produced by fatty acids in the blood or urine.

Ketones are a very efficient source of energy, so fasting is a wonderful way to lose weight, improve insulin, fight off depression, and boost brain functions. Most importantly, natural human growth hormone (HGH) increases, which is important for muscle growth, energy, and longevity when it is secreted naturally.

Research into Fasting and Longevity

In the 1930s, Clive McCay, a biochemist and gerontologist, put his lab rats on a low-calorie, high-protein, high-vitamin diet. McCay and his researchers found that the rats not only had lower rates of cancer but their lifespans increased by 20 to 50 percent. This effect was due to the lower energy consumed and not any other aspects of the diet. The science of calorie restriction (CR) was born. Hundreds of studies since McCay's success have shown that CR slows aging not only in mice and rats but also in yeast, flies, worms, and fish. It turned out that CR did not have to be continuous, in rats or in humans.

"Eat less often and in certain periods of the day" is now the new mantra of longevity experts. Experts went from saying, "Eat every three hours" to "eat only in eight hours." Intermittent fasting has a significant impact on longevity.

The impact of intermittent fasting on longevity on humans is unknown at this time. The positive findings are mostly from animal studies.

The Good News About Intermittent Fasting

Here is the good news about intermittent fasting: your body was built for it. Early humans endured fasting throughout most of their existence before the development of agriculture. You may not enjoy fasting at first, but, believe me, you have been genetically designed to succeed at periodic fasting. Like other mammals, tigers and lions do not eat for days until they find their next prey; we are no different. Being able to go without food for extended periods was essential to our survival. Adversity means a prolonged lifespan; comfort means early disease and death.

Think about it: back in the days when there was no such thing as food that was available year-round, being able to go without food was what separated those who would pass on their survival DNA to the next generation from those who would not. IF is more in keeping with our bodies' natural rhythms than eating three or more meals per day, often with snacks in between.

How to Practice Intermittent Fasting

The basic theory behind IF is to enjoy your meals at specific times of day, in a cyclical pattern of eating and not eating. That way, you will sharpen your ability to encourage longevity by getting rid of old proteins and old cells, also known as zombie cells. In turn, decreasing inflammation is achieved by getting rid of those old cells. You can slow down, and even reverse, some of the damage of unhealthy choices you made in the past.

Of course, there is a connection between *when* you eat and *what* you eat. You cannot fast for twenty-four hours and then eat a burger and some French fries and think that is going to have a positive health effect. You must use common sense to reap the benefits of IF. Maybe that's why some human studies on intermittent fasting showed negative results. You do not have to be overly restrictive, eat only a plant-based diet, or completely forgo treats or alcohol, but you do have to keep an eye on nutrition. You still need your body to function at its best while you are challenging it with IF stress.

There is more than one way to approach IF. Deciding which fasting is right for you, the right periods of fasting time, and sticking to the principles are the prime rules of successful fasting.

Here are some popular intermittent fasting plans.

- **The 16/8 method, or the Leangains protocol.** This is by far the most popular way to practice IF. It is also the easiest. If it is the approach that appeals to you most, you will be skipping breakfast and doing all your eating during an eight-hour window that begins in the afternoon. You might eat between 9 AM and 5 PM or 12 to 8 PM or 1 to 9 PM. If you eat breakfast, then eat a late lunch and skip dinner. Some research indicates that eating during the day is better to control weight. It makes sense since human growth hormone (HGH), a fat-burning hormone, is secreted at night and inhibited by food. If you eat a late dinner, it is not good for the secretion of HGH. Research from Spain shows more weight loss can be reached when you eat during the day and when your last meal is around 4 or 5 PM. Whatever works for you.

Just make sure that once you have finished your scheduled eating in eight hours, you do not eat a morsel until sixteen hours have passed. You can drink water or unsweetened tea in the sixteen hours of fasting time. There is some research that indicates this type of fast increases human mortality, but I believe this research is flawed as it goes against all positive findings in animal studies. People usually give poor history with their dietary habits. They also may eat the wrong things like fried foods after such prolonged fasts. If you do it every day, of course you may eat less nutrients and damage your body. But if it is done periodically, no one dies from skipping a meal.

- **Eat-Stop-Eat.** This method is straightforward and requires little recordkeeping or paying attention to the clock. It is, however, much more challenging. The "eat-stop-eat" plan requires you to fast for a full day or more! This means eating absolutely nothing for twenty-four hours or even longer. Some people go on this fast for a few days. You must do these twenty-four-hour fasts one or two times a month, depending on how you find your body reacting to those intervals. Although this is a tough one, this type of fasting may have the biggest impact on longevity as it has the most impact on many of the hallmarks of aging. You can drink water. If you fast for more than twenty-four hours, you will need to add electrolytes to your water. I did this fast once for forty-eight hours. Surprisingly, after the first twenty-four hours, my hunger pain went away. This is indeed an extreme form of fasting but early humans often survived without food for extended periods of time. Today, some biohackers do this type of prolonged fast regularly. However, I do not recommend doing this fast frequently as you can lose muscle mass.
- **The 5:2 method.** You eat an extremely limited number of calories on two nonconsecutive days, and, on the other five days of the week, you eat normal, healthy meals of reasonable calories. Basically, it is just cutting calories. On the days that you are eating limited calories, your

target should be no more or less than 500–600 calories for the day. Research done on animals and mice showed cutting calories on certain days led to weight loss but did not lead to a prolonged lifespan. So I do not advocate this type of fasting unless your goal is to lose weight.

I do a variety of intermittent fasting. Sometimes I eat a fat-rich breakfast at 8 AM and a late lunch at 4 PM. Sometimes, I skip breakfast and just do lunch and dinner. When I eat breakfast, I go for an omelet with cheese, or a keto coffee. I eat nothing after 4 or 5 PM. Having a fat-rich breakfast can help you succeed in staying hunger free for a long time. Sometimes, I reduce my caloric intake on certain days.

Summary of the Three Types of Fast

- Eating from 9 AM to 4 PM or 1 PM to 8 PM
- Eating just once a day or every few days
- Cutting calories on certain days

Liquids Allowed on Intermittent Fasting (IF)

No matter which plans of intermittent fasting you choose—eating only in eight-hour periods, eating nothing for twenty-four hours or more, or eating fewer calories on certain few days—remember to drink lots of liquids, as long as they are noncaloric. Again, add electrolytes; water, tea, decaf coffee, and mineral water are all good options. Drinking tea all day is fine if no sugar is added. Seltzer water is okay if you do not have heartburn. Keeping your stomach full of water will keep you hydrated.

Drinking liquids will prevent you from getting dizzy in the period when you are not eating. It is not necessary, but it is best to drink spring, glacial, or mineral water because they contain natural minerals.

Go for Nuts to Curb Hunger

If you *really* feel that you need something solid in your tummy during the fast, eat a few nuts. I mean a small handful of unsalted raw almonds, walnuts, ca-shews, or any nuts you like. Do not eat them in one or two mouthfuls. Instead, eat just a few at a time, then wait twenty minutes. You will find your hunger will disappear because even a small amount of natural, unprocessed food will satisfy you.

How to Succeed on a Fast

There can be many moments during a fast when you'll feel tempted to eat. Distract yourself by doing any activity that demands your complete atten-tion. Working on something that keeps your hands occupied is a good way to keep you from reaching for a snack—that would break your fast, and you would feel defeated. Writing, knitting, gardening, washing your car, or even brushing your teeth may help. So does physical exercise. Go for a walk, go to the gym, or play a sport. Even take a nap—you get the idea.

How Often to Fast

Try fasting once a week. You can eventually do it twice a week or more. Intermittent fasting can easily be done on weekends by going for brunch and dinner without interruption to your routine or your family. You could have tea in the morning and go for brunch at 1 PM. Easy. If you do more than a seventy-two-hour fast, do it on a Thursday as the fatigue will hit you two days later. The energy will not come before Sunday, or seventy-two hours later. You will have more chances to succeed if you are not at work. It isn't easy, but your body will adjust to this new way of eating. But I truly do not recommend this extreme form of fasting. Life is meant to be enjoyed. What's the point of living a long life, but hungry?

Things to Consider when Practicing IF

Each person is different, so you need to consider your work, family situation, obligations, and daily routines before you decide to try an IF plan. It's also es-sential to consult your doctor if you have any chronic illness such as diabetes because doses of medications must be adjusted down during the fasting periods or if you have an eating disorder.

Extended Fasts Can Be Dangerous

Although skipping meals for a few days may have the longest impact on longevity, extended fasts can become dangerous. Go to YouTube and watch the experience of some biohackers who have gone without food, and only water, for several weeks. They claim that their energy levels go up in three days because of ketone bodies, which you learned about earlier in this chapter and the effect they have on the brain-derived neurotrophic factor (BDNF) that goes up. But if you do not have fat reserves, you will start to lose muscle mass. You may get dizzy and faint. Again, I *do not* advocate this extreme approach. Moderation is key.

The Many Health Benefits of Intermittent Fasting

Don't be deterred by the idea of fasting. It's not easy, but you and your body will adjust if you start slowly and do it in moderation according to the guidelines in this chapter. You will see that the effect of IF on your health and improved longevity makes it a worthwhile practice. Here is a recap of the main benefits of IF:

- **Insulin resistance.** Intermittent fasting can reduce insulin resistance, lowering blood sugar by 3 to 6 percent and insulin levels by 20 to 31 percent, which is protective against type 2 diabetes.
- **Inflammation.** Some studies show reductions in inflammation markers, a key driver of many chronic diseases and aging.
- **Heart health.** Intermittent fasting may also reduce bad, small LDL cholesterol and blood triglycerides—both risk factors for heart disease.
- **Fights cancer.** Animal studies suggest that intermittent fasting may lower cancer risk.
- **Brain health.** Intermittent fasting increases the brain hormone BDNF and may aid the growth of new nerve cells. This may protect against Alzheimer's disease.

- **Anti-aging.** Intermittent fasting can extend lifespan in rats. Studies showed that fasting rats lived 36 to 50 percent longer. Although there is not sufficient data about the effects of IF on human lifespan, researchers agree that it is reasonable to induce a similar result for human subjects.

What to Eat After IF

So far, you've learned *how* you should eat (or not) during fasting, but not what you should eat after you've completed a fasting period. To keep it simple, it's no different from what I recommend you eat routinely. Focus on eating clean. This means whole, natural organic foods, and avoiding sugar, refined grains, preservatives, processed foods, and chemicals.

Like heart disease, cancer is the leading cause of death from aging. Nearly 2 million cases of cancer were diagnosed in 2022. The risk increases with each decade, and now cancer is affecting more young people. If this trend continues, cancer will account for more than a third of all deaths in people between ages forty-five and sixty-four. Eating clean, avoiding sugar, and intermittent fasting should be some of our weapons in this new way to age. With all the positive findings on IF, I would say, there's a new way to age.

Remember . . .

- Start slow. After you have skipped a meal, try to go for a longer fast.

- *When* you eat is as important as what you eat, so intermittent fasting should be part of your routine.

- Choose a fast you can follow on a regular basis. Do it a few times a month depending on your lifestyle and health.

- *Leangains protocol* entails not eating anything for sixteen hours, then eating only within an eight-hour period you choose. Always have dinner early, like at 5 or 6 PM.

- *The eat-stop-eat approach* might be the most challenging. You eat nothing for a full twenty-four-hour period or longer. This type of fasting has the most impact on longevity.

- *The 5:2 method* requires you to eat only 500–600 calories per day for two consecutive days. Eat regular, healthy meals on the other five days of the week. This type of fast makes you lose weight, but it has no impact on longevity.

- Never eat a late dinner.

- Breaking a fast: (1) Eat vegetables, low-sugar fruits, beans, lentils, whole grains, lean protein, and healthy fats. (2) While fasting, let your body burn fat between meals. Do not snack. (3) Stay busy and exercise to build muscle. (4) Drink a lot of water to stay hydrated and fill your stomach.

- Eat adequate amounts of protein during IF.

- Stay active during fast and exercise so you do not lose muscle mass.

- Check out examples of different types of fasting days in the Appendix.

CHAPTER 15

Having an Ageless Body and Mind

Difficulties strengthen the mind,
as labor does the body.
—**Seneca**

IF everyone maintained *a healthy weight, did not smoke, and exercised regularly, they would live long, healthy, vigorous lives. But often, many people eat poorly, don't exercise, and even smoke, which can mean living ten to twenty years with age-related diseases culminating in a painful death with a lot of suffering. Exercise can make a big difference when it comes to staying healthier longer. But how does exercise actually impact longevity? It's thanks to the hormetic stress effect on sirtuins, the CEO of your cells.*

Bad Stress and Good Stress: Why It Matters

Stress can play havoc with your body and mind. Bad stress is linked to anxiety, feeling overwhelmed, and pressured by major responsibilities. This is the type of stress you always want to avoid if you are on your journey to your best health and longest life! It shortens your telomeres and stunts your stem cells.

But hormetic stress is a good stress. It is good for you. It actually strengthens your cells and improves health and longevity.

Hormetic, or good, stress is your best friend. It triggers your sirtuins, the signaling and longevity proteins.

What Exactly Is Hormetic Stress and How Does It Work?

Hormetic stress, also known as hormesis, is how cells respond and adapt when they are intermittently exposed to low levels of stress. This type of stress produces certain kinds of proteins like restorative growth factors and antioxidant enzymes. Those are the same proteins that help us repair damaged and diseased cells, and even prevent our cells from being susceptible to damage in the first place. This kind of cell activity is the secret weapon in all of our anti-aging efforts.

A limited and controlled amount of stress of a very particular kind, plus rest, equals growth. You can elicit a positive chemical response within your body if you expose yourself to mild levels of stressors. Hormetic stress has been well researched and proven to be an effective way to stave off disease, fight aging, and prevent early death.

Creating Hormetic Stress

There are several ways that you can create hormetic stress to get these benefits. The methods I have found easiest to incorporate into the average person's lifestyle are intermittent fasting and exercise.

Exercise can dramatically alter your health and longevity right down to the cellular level. You can significantly alter both your quality of life and your lifespan this way. No matter who you are or what you do for your daily routine, you will always benefit from simply moving your body. It exercises your heart, improves circulation, and lowers your insulin levels.

Easy Ways to Incorporate Exercise into Your Day

The good news is that you don't have to spend hours at the gym or the track to get exercise. Start with common daily activities. Here are some simple ways to incorporate exercise into your daily life without much effort:

- Make it a habit to take the stairs instead of the elevator or escalator all the time. Walk to the corner store instead of driving.

- If you take a bus or subway, get off one stop before your destination and walk the rest of the way.

- When you do have to drive, park your car as far away from your destination as possible to force yourself to walk.

- Wash your car by hand instead of taking it to the car wash.

- Watching TV? Walk or jog in place or lift light weights (water bottles will do!) instead of sitting down. Also, skip the remote and get up to change the channel.

- Add a ten-minute walk to your lunch break or coffee break at work.

- Using the phone? Stand up and stretch or pace during the call.

- At work, use the bathroom on a different floor and take the stairs.

- Walk your dog daily. They need the exercise and bonding experience as much as you do, and you'll have the added benefit of getting to know your other dog-walking neighbors!

Daily activities can easily become good habits that you will soon find yourself doing automatically. People who live in the Blue Zones make exercise part of their daily lives. They don't go to expensive gyms or wear fitness trackers to ensure they get 10,000 steps each day.

The Three Types of Exercise

There are three types of exercise: aerobic, anaerobic, and high-intensity interval training (HIIT). Whatever exercise you choose to do, it will still be good for your health. All forms of exercise will challenge you in separate ways. Exercise gives you benefits by working on sirtuins 1 and 3.

When you exercise, your body also releases feel-good endorphins. Popular culture identifies these as the chemicals behind "runner's high," a short-lasting euphoric state following intense exercise. Exercise also improves insulin levels. Research shows that a newly discovered hormone called irisin protects against metabolic diseases such as diabetes. Whatever your age,

exercise should be part of your lifestyle.

Talk to Your Doctor Before Starting a New Exercise Routine
As with any new exercise routine, talk to your doctor first before starting, especially if you have been a couch potato, have a chronic condition, or are over fifty. Start slow.

Aerobic Exercise

Aerobic means "with oxygen." Aerobic exercise relies on the energy stored in your body from carbs, proteins, fat, and the oxygen you breathe. You can do aerobic exercise for short, moderate, or extended periods of time.

During aerobic exercise, your breathing and heart rate increase for an extended period, increasing blood flow to the muscles and back to the lungs as you move large muscles in your arms, legs, and hips and maximize the amount of oxygen in your blood.

Aerobic exercise strengthens bones and burns fat. While increasing your stamina, it reduces the risk of type 2 diabetes, heart attacks, and stroke. Since it boosts your immune system, colds and flu are less frequent. It also produces endorphins, which boost your mood. It is great for weight loss.

Aerobic exercise is excellent for cardiovascular conditioning and improving muscular endurance. Studies have shown that aerobic exercise improves estrogen metabolism in women. Think brisk walks, water aerobics, tennis, swimming laps, bike riding, jogging, or sweating through a Zumba class. Choose something you like to do so you'll stick with it. The American Heart Association recommends healthy adults get at least thirty minutes of aerobic exercise at least five days a week.

Anaerobic Exercise

Anaerobic means "without oxygen," such as lifting weights. This type of exercise leads to increased secretion of human growth hormone (HGH). This helps build muscles and prevents osteoporosis.

Anaerobic exercise entails short, fast, high-intensity exercise of lifting weights, a short rest period, and another period of exercise. This type of exercise burns glucose in your muscles for energy. During anaerobic exercise, your muscles exert maximum force in short intervals of time with the goal of not only increasing power but also building better oxygen use.

Anaerobic exercise produces restorative growth factors and antioxidant enzymes, the same proteins that repair damaged cells and protect our cells. This type of cell activity is the secret ingredient to all anti-aging efforts. This type of exercise can help prevent Alzheimer's disease. Lifting weights can also help improve testosterone production in men. A limited and controlled amount of stress of a very particular kind, plus rest for muscles, equals growth.

High-Intensity Interval Training (HIIT)

High-intensity interval training (HIIT) is the toughest form of exercise, but it also has the greatest impact on longevity. Imagine exercising so hard that you have to stop to catch your breath, and you can hardly talk or say your name. It is very tough. However, you can increase your progress in small increments, at your own pace until you reach that stage. As you go along, you will feel better and better and *want* to do more. How to do it? Push yourself to the limit until you lose your breath and need a break. Repeat. Imagine that you are running from a bear in the forest.

HIIT is proven to deliver health results far beyond the average trip to the gym for an aerobics class or lifting weights. The goal of HIIT is to tax your body with exercise to push your cardiovascular and muscular endurance to its limits for short bursts of time, followed by rest or active recovery, followed by more cycles of intense exercise. Doing this for about fifteen minutes—or less for beginners—brings plenty of rewards. HIIT can stave off disease and extend your lifespan by up to a decade.

In one session, HIIT can reduce blood pressure, and if you develop a steady habit of HIIT exercise, it will reduce the risk of cardiovascular disease. As you become consistent in your routine, it will feel easier than slow training programs.

HIIT significantly increases volume oxygen max (VO2 max), the highest amount of oxygen you can use during an intense workout. The higher your VO2 max, the more energy your body uses, and the longer you can exercise. Research shows that those who used HIIT had a greater excess post-exercise oxygen consumption (EPOC), the amount of oxygen needed for homeostasis, than those who did steady-rate exercise.

HIIT is the gift that keeps on giving. After exercising this way, you will continue to burn calories throughout the day to reoxygenate your blood and cool down your core temperature. Your body is restoring itself to homeostasis—your normal metabolic state. You are using more oxygen to replenish adenosine triphosphate (ATP)—the energy-carrying molecules in the cells of all living things—that you used working out.

Target Heart Rate Matters

When you increase your heart rate, you improve your circulation. You get the full benefits of exercise. According to the CDC, for vigorous-intensity physical activity, your target heart rate should be between 77 and 93 percent of your maximum heart rate. To calculate your maximum heart rate, subtract your age from 220. For example, for a thirty-five-year-old person, the estimated maximum age-related heart rate would be calculated as 220 − 35 years = 185 beats per minute (bpm). The 77 percent level is 185 × 0.77 = 142 bpm, and the 93 percent level is 185 × 0.93 = 172 bpm. For this thirty-five-year-old, the optimal heart rate range is 142 bpm to 172 bpm during a workout. Of course, no matter your age, consult with your doctor before starting any type of exercise routine, especially one as strenuous as HIIT.

Strengthen Your Bones

One of the biggest challenges we face as we get older is bone loss. As a result, we can get fractures. As we age, the bones become brittle and weak. This happens as women lose estrogen and men lose testosterone. From the outside, the bones look normal, but from the inside, they are porous. Often the person will sustain a fracture from a mild trauma. Prevention is key. Anaerobic exercise and running are great.

Low vitamin D, calcium deficiency, smoking, and excess alcohol can all contribute to bone loss. Consuming high-calcium food is essential. So take vitamin D3 5000 IU a day. Also take calcium citrate 500 mg at least two to three times a day. It is also important to take vitamin K2 when you take calcium so the calcium gets deposited in the bones and not in your coronary arteries. If you want tangible results or have significant bone loss, look into OsteoStrong; the company produced this unique system. OsteoStrong provides a unique system for strengthening joints, bones, and muscles by using a process called osteogenic loading. During each session, you will utilize a series of devices that allow axial compression of bone to emulate the effect of impact—that means pressure on your bones will be simulated in a way that avoids any damage. Because of the optimized positioning of the human body, loading forces go through the human bones that are far higher than those seen in daily activity or weight training. Yes, this program costs money, like expensive gyms, but it does not have to be the only way to build strong bones. You can always do anaerobic exercise on your own, and it would not cost you a thing.

Exercise Your Brain on *The Ageless Revolution*

The human brain is truly a mind-boggling and complex organ. It is composed of neurons that generate enough electricity to charge a cell phone in seventy hours. If your brain were Netflix or Hulu, you would have enough storage to watch streaming shows nonstop for three centuries. However, one in ten people over the age of sixty-five has some form of dementia, so prevention is key. Bad protein starts to accumulate in the brain ten to twenty years before the onset of the symptoms of Alzheimer's disease. We also lose neurons as we age, but new research shows we can generate new brain cells in our sixties, seventies, and even eighties.

To have a healthy brain and generate new brain cells, you need good blood circulation and good nutrients. Exercise improves circulation and can help with brain fog. The brain is mostly made of fat, so eat more healthy fats, such as the ones found in fish and seafood. Also eat more berries, which are rich in antioxidants, and avoid or limit sugar.

Give your brain a workout every day. New tasks challenge the brain. Learn a new language or learn a new word every day. Do crosswords or play chess. I challenge my brain by learning new languages, novel words, reading research studies, and learning about art and history. Stress is very bad for brain health. So it is also important to get rid of negative thoughts as it can lead to negative brain health. Stress can kill brain cells and reduce the size of the brain.

A Patient's Story

Brandon, fifty-two, insisted he did not have time to exercise. He was not obese but had put on a few pounds and said that no matter how much he dieted he just could not take it off. He felt tired and sluggish and was starting to feel a little depressed. He had joined a gym a year earlier, went twice, hated it, and never went back. Plus, he said his schedule was too busy for two-hour workouts three or four times a week. That was his problem!

No one can go from never working out to spending six or eight hours at the gym! I suggested he take small steps instead. Literally! His office at work was on the third floor, and he started to take the stairs each day. I also encouraged him just to go for short walks—on his coffee break, after dinner, whenever he could. When he ran errands, he parked as far from the store as possible so he would walk a little more. He started lifting some light weights whenever he watched TV. Bonus: that stopped him from snacking!

These were minor steps, but they added up. He lost ten pounds over the next three months and began feeling like he had more energy. Gradually, we increased his exercise, and he took longer walks and occasional jogs and started using heavier weights. Now he is ready to give the gym another go.

Like Brandon, it is important to start slow, and take baby steps. I do not expect you to do HIIT if you have been a couch potato. With exercise, you're optimizing the nutrient pathways, you are burning excess calories, you are repairing your cells, and you are fighting muscle loss. You are on your way to becoming ageless.

Remember . . .

- *Hormetic stress* is stress that is good for you. It is a limited and controlled amount of stress of a very particular kind.
- If you have no time to work out, exercise on weekends.
- *Aerobic* exercise is less intense, so you can continue to breathe through your routine for a longer period.
- *Anaerobic* exercise means "without oxygen." Be careful. Start with low weights.
- *HIIT* requires you to use your muscles to exert maximum force in short intervals, then cool down for a brief period, and start again, repeating for fifteen minutes. You keep going until you can hardly breathe; you have no more air. HIIT has the most impact on longevity.
- *HIIT* increases cardiovascular and muscle endurance and lowers blood pressure and heart disease risks. It burns more calories after you finish the workout because your body takes longer to return to its normal metabolic rate.
- *Consult your doctor* before you start any type of exercise, especially HIIT.
- Exercise your brain. You need a sharp mind as you get older.
- Stay motivated. *Remember the benefits of exercise for the body and brain for longevity.*

CHAPTER 16

Turn Back Time with the Right Supplements

Instead of asking a doctor to prescribe me a drug when I'm ill, I'd rather take something that can help me avoid getting sick in the first place.
—**Laird Hamilton**

People who cracked the longevity code in the five Blue Zones eat natural food, live a stress-free life, and remain active. It is that simple. Many folks in these areas become centenarians. But can humans live to 110 or 120 years? I do not see a reason why this cannot be achieved if we target our cells. So let us conquer the ten hallmarks of aging like those folks naturally or like the super rich, but on a budget. It is time to attack the cellular deterioration full force and with an arsenal of weapons. Or as I call them, the right supplements that can turn back time. Do we need supplements? No. But I think of supplements as a form of insurance. They can cover shortfalls in diet, exercise, and lifestyle.

Supplements need to be an important part of your arsenal when it comes to healthy living and longevity. According to a 2019 poll by the American

Osteopathic Association, 86 percent of Americans take supplements. But which supplement will make you live longer?

A meta-analysis from Johns Hopkins found out that only two supplements can make us live longer: folic acid and omega-3 fatty acids. Taking omega-3 fatty acids is linked to living longer because it improves heart health and reduces heart attacks by 10 percent by fighting inflammation. Taking folic acid at an older age has been controversial. But does this mean other supplements can't target the ten hallmarks of aging? No. But there are simply no human studies on most of these supplements and longevity.

Most of the supplements I recommend here have been tested on animals with positive results on their aging process, so hopefully, they will help us too. Human studies are ongoing. It is important that you consult with your personal physician before starting a supplement regimen.

The World of Supplements: What You Need to Know

Go to any health food or vitamin store, or even a chain supermarket or drugstore, and you will find an aisle labeled "supplements" with a wide range of pills, capsules, lotions, chewable gummies, and liquids. Supplements are intended to boost the efficacy of whatever else you are already eating, like adding nutrients that may be missing from your diet. Most supplements are vitamins, synthetic versions of chemicals that are naturally produced by your body.

But which supplement succeeded in fighting cellular aging in animal studies? Which supplement will make you live longer? There are hundreds, if not thousands, of supplements that are labeled with anti-aging claims. Very few of these products are regulated by the FDA or any other medical advisory board. There is no need for a prescription, no advice beyond when in the day to take them, and no information about the full effects of what you are taking. It is up to you to do the research. Few people do. Don't worry. I have reviewed the research studies for you, which will make it easy for you to know what to take. Most over-the-counter supplements won't make a difference to your health despite what the labels may say. But some do. The right supplements act on your genes and cells, which will improve your ability to live a significantly longer and healthier life. Those are the supplements that scientists in the anti-aging area are looking into.

Fish Oil

There is no doubt that people with higher omega-3 fatty acids lived longer than people with lower levels, with an increased life expectancy of 4.7 years. Some people may notice improvement in as little as four to eight weeks. Fish oil helps with cardiovascular health and skin. Some doctors say krill oil, which comes from crustaceans, is superior to fish oil, but more research is needed. Some people are allergic to fish, but the allergy is mostly related to the protein, not the oil. Take 1 gram a day.

Taurine

I truly love this supplement. In a population study spanning twenty-five countries and more than 14,000 people, scientists found that residents of Okinawa in Japan, one of the five Blue Zones, had the *highest* intake of taurine along with the *lowest* rate of heart disease and the *longest* average lifespan. In animal studies, taking taurine extends longevity by 25 percent. What does this mean for us humans? It means, taking taurine can probably extend your life by four to eight years. Taurine is a low-cost amino acid found in diet that facilitates a diverse range of biological functions. Evidence suggests that *increasing* taurine supply may have potential benefits for cardiovascular disorders, high cholesterol, and Alzheimer's disease. It improves heart health, energizes the mitochondria, stimulates stem cell production, helps repair DNA, and extends lifespans. Research published in the medical journal *Science* showed that older adults suffer a dramatic decrease in levels of taurine. This decline means more rapid aging and increased rates of age-related diseases. To counteract this decrease and maintain higher taurine levels, eat the right foods and/or supplement with this important nutrient. Dietary sources of taurine include seafood like scallops, mussels, and clams. Dark meat in chicken, and turkey are also good sources of taurine. But it can be challenging to obtain this amount of taurine from food alone. Most successful clinical studies with taurine have used daily doses of 1500 mg to 3000 mg. I used to take 500 mg a long time ago, but I upped the dose to 2 grams a day. A word of caution: Taurine acts like a diuretic, meaning it can drop your blood pressure; it's important to have it checked before you take this supplement. I have placed taurine as one of the top supplements to consider in *The Ageless Revolution*.

Fisetin

Fisetin is a senolytic that kills the old cells and reduces the senescent cells (zombie cells) burden that can accumulate with age or disease. Senolytics are a class of drugs that kill the old or senescent cells. Intermittent fasting kills the zombie cells too. But who can starve all the time? Fisetin does that job, so it fits the bill.

Didn't I promise to make *The Ageless Revolution* easy and doable for you? Fisetin is found in certain foods such as apples and strawberries. But it's impossible to eat enough of those fruits to gain benefit from fisetin, so supplementation may be necessary.

Fisetin in combination with healthy lifestyle choices can create a potent combination that could reduce the pathological processes of aging, potentially yielding positive effects on both health span and lifespan.

Currently, fisetin dosage and frequency suggestions for longevity are unknown. We do not have human studies on fisetin. Animal studies are very promising. Fisetin research is still in its infancy, but it should be prioritized in the battle against the zombie cells. One study done on mice in 2018 showed that removing senescent cells made the mice live 36 percent longer than mice that did not have senescent cells removed. I prefer you do intermittent fasting than taking fisetin. If you decide to take fisetin, the dose is 500 mg a day.

Pterostilbene

Pterostilbene is the newest kid on the block for anti-aging because it activates sirtuins that repair DNA. Pterostilbene and its famous brother, resveratrol, are similar natural molecules found in fruits, vegetables, and nuts. But resveratrol breaks down quickly in the body while pterostilbene is much better in terms of absorption and stability. Pterostilbene is a natural molecule found in vegetables, fruits, and nuts. Yes, you can eat an enormous number of blueberries if you want, but you won't get enough pterostilbene to have an influence in your life. We also do not have human studies on pterostilbene and longevity. Pterostilbene can help brain function and can activate the AMPK pathway, which protects the cells from aging. Recommended dose of pterostilbene is 150 mg a day.

Resveratrol

Resveratrol turns on the CEO of your cells: sirtuins. This compound is found in red wine and may explain the French paradox. Researchers studied this and took a closer look at the traditional French diet, which consists of copious amounts of animal products (foie gras, escargots, boeuf bourguignon) and the remarkably small number of heart attacks, strokes, and other diseases experienced by other populations. Could it be the butter, walking, or the red wine?

Some researchers claim that the red wine that the French typically drink with meals is the key to health and longevity. That's because the resveratrol in red wine is a powerful antioxidant. Resveratrol is also found in a variety of foods such as blueberries, bilberries (smaller and darker than blueberries), cranberries, peanuts, and cocoa.

Not only does resveratrol sweep free radicals from the body, but it is also believed to prevent a multitude of diseases, including various forms of cancer, cardiovascular disease, degenerative brain disease, and ailments created by continuous inflammation.

Many animal studies on resveratrol were controversial, and the benefits were not replicated. Some even argue that high doses of resveratrol may be toxic. All this is unknown. If you wish to add resveratrol to your regimen, I recommend taking one gram of trans-resveratrol daily in a white powder form with full-fat organic yogurt for maximal absorption. Do not take it if it is yellow. Hopefully, we can have more research in the near future. It isn't on my preferred list.

Quercetin

Quercetin is another senolytic, which means it can selectively eliminate senescent or old cells, one of the ten hallmarks of aging. Senescent cells or zombie cells can't divide any longer and release inflammatory molecules that interfere with the function of healthy cells. Quercetin, a plant chemical, or flavonoid, has antioxidant properties that neutralize free radicals, which damage DNA, and reduce inflammation by removing senescent cells. You have heard the saying "Eating an apple a day keeps the doctor away." Could it be because they contain quercetin? Research also shows that quercetin, not caffeine, in coffee is the primary compound that is responsible for the drink's potential protective effects against Alzheimer's. Quercetin is also found in teas, onions, apples, buckwheat, red wine, and berries, in purple foods like eggplant, and in green foods like broccoli and kale. If you decide to take quercetin, the dose is 500–1000 mg daily.

Nicotinamide Adenine Dinucleotide (NAD)

Nicotinamide adenine dinucleotide, or NAD, is another supplement on the top of my list to consider. Buzz has been steadily growing around a tiny molecule with immense potential in anti-aging; it is called nicotinamide adenine dinucleotide, also known as NAD. Why? Sirtuins require NAD to function.

It is a no-brainer that NAD may slow the aging process—giving it the title "the fountain of youth supplement." NAD, a crucial coenzyme found in every cell of the body that boosts metabolism, plays a central role in various biological processes, including energy production, DNA repair, and regulation of gene expression. As we age, NAD levels decline. Hollywood celebrities are flocking to clinics and doctors now to get NAD drips and injections. NAD not only works on sirtuins, but it also helps repair the DNA and works on mitochondria as well, the battery of our cells. Remember how much energy you had when you were young? You bounced out of bed quickly, feeling rejuvenated and ready to take on every day like a champion. That was when your cells worked to their fullest potential thanks in large part to the mitochondria, which are energy powerhouses. They generate approximately 90 percent of your energy and are essential for organ function and sustaining life.

Unfortunately, our mitochondria get damaged as we age, causing our cells to lose power. Low levels of NAD lead the cells to work less efficiently. How much to take? NAD levels can be measured by a test, but the test is not widely available.

The physical benefits of NAD therapy are impressive. NAD is sometimes called a "helper molecule" because it binds with other enzymes and helps them do their job better. NAD optimizes brain function, and supports cardiovascular and muscle health, speeds recovery from injury, and improves metabolism and immune function. NAD helps detox because it lessens withdrawal symptoms and diminishes cravings for harmful substances. It even improves eyesight and hearing, helps weight loss, decreases pain, and protects nerves. Now that we know how important NAD is, what form do we take?

When you look for NAD supplements, you will find NAD, NAD+, and NADH sold in stores. In general terms, they are all NAD, but processed in the body differently or are a molecule that can form it inside our body.

For your body to make NAD, it requires a precursor. Think of it this way, you need building materials to build a house, like wood and steel. The same goes for NAD. The supplements that are precursors to NAD include nicotinamide riboside (NR), nicotinamide mononucleotide (NMN), nicotinic acid

(NA), nicotinamide (NAM), tryptophan (TRP), and nicotinamide phosphoribosyl transferase (NAMPT). You can take a precursor or take NAD. But what will give the optimal results? NAD is a large molecule and difficult to absorb intracellularly. So even if you take NAD through IV drips or through a skin patch, it may not even boost NAD adequately since it is not absorbed very well. So it is better to take a precursor such as NMN or NR. Taking both NR and NMN offers maximal benefits. In one study, elderly mice given a precursor called nicotinamide riboside experienced a 5 percent increase in lifespan. For humans, this means possibly four years of longevity.

Unfortunately, the FDA banned the sale of NMN during the writing of this book even though animal studies show its benefits. Instead, take 300 mg a day of NR daily. If you find NMN online from overseas, take one gram a day. It's definitely better to take both (NR and NMN). Whatever way you decide to take, or find online, it would be better to take NR than nothing.

If you decide to take NAD as a drip at your doctor's office, that process gets NAD directly into your bloodstream rather than being degraded in the stomach when NAD is taken orally. But NAD drips are quite expensive and take two to three hours to administer. The process must also be repeated every one to two weeks for the anti-aging benefits. This could run you $800 a drip, so a precursor like NR; it is much cheaper and will do the anti-aging job to get your NAD levels up. I must say that some research indicates that NR may increase breast cancer risk, but this is still elusive.

Trimethyglycine (TMG)

Trimethyglycine, also known as betaine, is an important antioxidant that the body can produce itself. It is involved in a chemical process called methylation, which is essential to the production of neurotransmitters and other biological functions. While taking NAD, it is also important to take trimethyglycine (TMG) along with it, as NAD needs a partner. TMG is a type of betaine, a chemical compound that helps correct improper digestion and hormonal disruptions. As your body uses NAD+, it gets broken down into waste that needs to be excreted from the body. To do this, we need a methyl group; that's when TMG comes into play. The more NAD+ supplements you take, the faster your methyl groups are depleted. TMG can be an important supplement on the days you take an NAD precursor to help with the chemical equation. TMG may also lower homocysteine levels, a protein that has been linked to heart attacks when extremely high.

Homocysteine levels rise with both high protein/low-carb and keto diets, since they are rich in animal products. Many athletes use TMG supplements with the aim of improving their athletic ability and enhancing exercise performance.

Several studies have found that TMG supplements may also improve insulin resistance, a condition that impairs your body's ability to use the hormone insulin to regulate blood sugar levels. In an animal study, administering TMG supplements to mice on a high-fat diet improved fat metabolism and decreased insulin resistance. The most common side effects associated with TMG supplements are digestive issues that include diarrhea, indigestion, and bloating. Take 1–2 grams of TMG daily, and start slowly, especially if you take NAD.

Vitamin D

Vitamin D is really a hormone and plays a huge role in overall health and wellness. It keeps our bones and immune system strong and much, much more. Vitamin D is a true anti-aging vitamin, and it serves every part of your body. For example, vitamin D helps maintain cognitive function as we age. People with Alzheimer's disease, brain fog, and any form of memory decline have low levels of vitamin D. Vitamin D has significant neuroprotective effects, including clearing amyloid plaques, a hallmark of Alzheimer's disease.

However, vitamin D is essential at every stage of life, starting with brain development in the womb, to decrease the risk for learning and memory problems. Severe problems for children born to vitamin D-deficient mothers include hypoxic-ischemic brain injury and the risk for autism, schizophrenia, and other mental illnesses later in life.

Vitamin D and Covid-19

Vitamin D played a huge role in minimizing the effect of Covid-19 infections by boosting the immune system. It reduced morbidity and mortality with Covid-19 infections severalfold. If your blood levels of vitamin D are over fifty, your chance of dying from Covid-19 is almost zero. Sadly, too many young people died during the Covid-19 pandemic because their vitamin D levels were simply too low, and their immune system was too weak. Living indoors with no sun exposure and following a low-fat diet made these young people very susceptible to the ravages of Covid-19. Their immune system was weak. It is sad that many families lost their loved ones unnecessarily. I saw the sadness, agony, and tears in their eyes as I tried to console them. So many people would have not died from Covid-19 if we followed the right precautions, like taking this important vitamin.

Vitamin D also inhibits inflammation and regulates white blood cells so that they can help heal the body. When it comes to fighting cardiovascular disease, cancer, diabetes, multiple sclerosis, infertility, and depression, vitamin D helps by cooling inflammation and boosting immune function. Vitamin D even reinforces the activation and growth of telomeres, the protective end caps on your chromosomes. This is important because as we age, telomeres shorten, and our DNA becomes unstable and prone to damage. When these cells die, this leads to oxidative stress, a major factor in aging. This increases the risk of liver disease, pulmonary fibrosis, gastrointestinal disease, bone marrow failure, and other problems.

On the cosmetic side, vitamin D plays a role in healthy skin aging. With a proper daily dose, vitamin D combats wrinkles and fine lines on the face.

The Sun and Vitamin D

In the twentieth century, experts thought that time in the sun was not advisable because of the risk of skin cancer, but moderate sun exposure for about twenty minutes a day is perfectly okay. In fact, we need it so the skin can manufacture the vitamin D we need to run so many processes in our body. But don't overdo it. If you are at the pool or the beach, take in some sun for twenty minutes, then cover yourself. Wear a big hat, sit under a giant umbrella, and use 50 SPF or higher sunscreen after your initial sun exposure. Make sure to stay away from sunscreen products containing parabens. I have already discussed the types of sunscreen you should use.

If you spend most of your time indoors, foods have negligible amounts of vitamin D. So a little bit of sun would be good for you. A glass of milk has only 100 IU of vitamin D. But it is found in salmon, herring, sardines, cod-liver oil, canned tuna, egg yolks, mushrooms, full-fat milk and yogurt.

You can also take vitamin D3 as a supplement along with its helper, calcium. Vitamin D boosts calcium absorption, which is essential for bone health and the prevention and treatment of osteoporosis.

Vitamin K2 also helps the body absorb vitamin D and direct calcium to your bones, not your arteries. Magnesium also improves vitamin D absorption.

So should you take vitamin D? It depends on where you live. Do you live in a sunny area, or a cloudy area in the northern hemisphere? If you live in a sunny arena, get some sun for twenty minutes a day. If you live in the northern hemisphere and don't have enough sun, take vitamin D3 at a dose of 5,000 to 10,000 IU a day with natural fats like nuts or fish oil to maximize absorption. But make sure not to overdo it. Vitamin D blood levels should be between 60 nmol/l to 80 nmol/l. If you take too much vitamin D3, you can end up with side effects related to vitamin D toxicity.

Spermidine

Spermidine, a naturally occurring molecule, is a fascinating compound and only now have researchers been able to understand it. Spermidine is part of a group of molecules known as polyamines that interact with our cells to perform a variety of metabolic functions. Spermidine is found in plants and animals and in nearly every cell of our body.

Loss of stable protein synthesis is one of the ten hallmarks of aging. This means that the protein in the cells is of poor quality, but the body can digest these bad proteins and products by a process called autophagy. Research indicates that spermidine has fascinating effects like fasting and recycling damaged cell components. Spermidine also regulates DNA stability, cellular growth, and cellular differentiation. Research in treating older mice with spermidine led to a decrease in arterial stiffening, which is an age-related condition correlated with deterioration of autophagy. Top spermidine foods are wheat germ, hazelnuts, cruciferous vegetables, soybeans, mushrooms, peas, chicken liver, cheddar cheese, and mangoes. You can eat these types of food, or you can take 1–2 mg of spermidine a day.

Astragalus Root

There are thousands of studies that show telomere shortening, a hallmark of aging, is related to poor health and a shorter life. To counteract this problem, scientists have developed new and innovative ways to activate an enzyme called telomerase with the use of astragalus root. This plant has been used in traditional Chinese medicine for centuries for longevity.

TA-65 is made through a proprietary process that increases astragalus absorption. It's expensive, starting at $100 for a bottle of thirty 100-unit capsules, and you will typically need to take between one and four capsules daily. There are other products on the market that cost less but they are less effective. Still, they can make a difference. TA-65 can be taken as fluid extract or pill form from 100 to 500 IU a day. Consult your doctor for the appropriate dosage for your size and age. If you take TA-65, you will be helping your cells stay young and healthy and you'll also notice that your dreams become vivid, and you'll sleep better. Selenium and ubiquinol are good substitutes for the high and prohibitive cost of TA-65. They are much cheaper, less than $20 a month. They are our best alternative options on *The Ageless Revolution*.

Selenium

Want longer telomeres? Think selenium. L-selenomethionine is a natural form of selenium found in plants. Dietary sources of selenium have minimal risk of overdose and are found in Brazil nuts, mushrooms, and many other fruits and vegetables such as broccoli and spinach. A new small study demonstrated that participants taking selenium at 200 mcg per day together with ubiquinol at 200 mg a day had longer telomeres and had five aging biomarkers that were significantly lower than in the placebo group.

Plasmalogens

Plasmalogens, extracted from sea squirts commonly eaten in Asian cuisines, are in the experimental stage for anti-aging. These fats are found in cell membranes and cell walls and decrease with age. However, recent research shows that taking plasmalogens as a supplement can reverse this and may reverse Alzheimer's disease.

Healthy cell walls ensure that cells can communicate effectively. Remember that impaired cellular communication is one of the ten hallmarks of aging. For the best results, take 0.5 mg for healthy individuals. A larger dose like 1 mg is recommended for people with existing brain disease.

Vitamin K2

Vitamin K2 was discovered in 1929 and does not receive much attention, but it plays an essential role in health. Vitamin K2 helps fight heart disease, the number one cause of mortality in the Western world. This helps prevent calcium from being deposited in your arteries.

People with the appropriate amount of vitamin K2 are less likely to have arterial calcification, heart disease, or osteoporosis. Vitamin K2 is found in fermented foods such as yogurt and traditional buttermilk, foods popular in the Blue Zones. Excess sugar and the official low-fat recommendations that were intended to prevent heart disease are doing the exact opposite! In fact, K2 is rare in Western diets because low-fat foods are promoted and eaten now, and we need natural fat in our diet to absorb this important fat-soluble vitamin. I take vitamin K2 at a dosage of 45 mcg daily.

Carnosine

Carnosine is a dipeptide that can delay aging and has been shown to rejuvenate aging cells in animal studies. Levels plummet as humans age, making supplementation a key part of an age-delaying program. Carnosine fights oxidation, mitochondrial dysfunction, and telomeres shortening. It preserves cognition and protects against heart disease. Take 500–2,000 mg of carnosine a day.

Glucosamine

Glucosamine is a natural molecule found in shellfish and in our cartilage and skin. It extends lifespan in multiple organisms because it can mimic a calorie-restricted diet. We don't know if glucosamine intake reduces mortality, but it does protect against DNA damage and reduce inflammation. It works against mitochondrial dysfunction, genomic or chromosome instability, and altered cell communications—three hallmarks of aging. Take 1,500 mg of glucosamine a day.

Calcium Alpha-Ketoglutarate

Three genes, OCT4, SOX2, and KLF4, or OSK for short, can reverse age by 60 to 75 percent. Calcium alpha-ketoglutarate is a molecule that is naturally present in the body and is activated before we are born to keep our stem cells healthy. As we age, levels go down.

However, these three genes, activated by calcium alpha ketoglutarate, can reverse our biological age. In mice, it extended lifespan by 12 percent. This molecule is also used as fuel by mitochondria, regulates the epigenome especially when taken with vitamin C, and supports stem cell health. Take one to two grams a day.

Berberine and Dihydroberberine (DHB)

Berberine is an alkaloid that occurs in various plants such as goldenseal, barberry, and Oregon grape. But berberine is not very well absorbed in the body. Dihydroberberine (DHB), a supplement, has a better absorption rate. Not only does it increase levels of glutathione to combat oxidative damage, but it may also prevent atherosclerosis and even heart failure because it improves blood flow to the heart. Through gut microbiota it decreases fat cell production and increases fat breakdown. DHB also reduces inflammation in the central nervous system, which can improve cognition, learning, and memory; ease anxiety and depression; and help prevent Parkinson's and Huntington's diseases. It may also help control blood sugar levels.

Dihydroberberine promotes longevity by activating AMPK, a pathway in the cells that regulate nutrient sensing, resulting in healthier cells and cellular longevity. AMPK levels reduce as we age. Supplement with 150 mg twice a day. Dihydroberberine can cause stomach issues when taken in substantial amounts over the recommended dose.

Methylene Blue

Methylene blue is a man-made medicine; it is not a natural supplement. But don't let the fact that methylene blue started out as a fabric dye in 1876 scare you. It has come a long way since then. It became the first manufactured synthetic medical treatment for malaria and gonorrhea; the antidote for the life-threatening condition methemoglobinemia, which prevents blood from reaching the tissues; and a treatment for the toxic effects of certain chemotherapy drugs as well as circulatory shock. It may also reduce cognitive decline, and offers pain relief. Methylene blue works on a cellular level on dysfunctional mitochondria (a hallmark of aging) to encourage energy production and subdue oxidative stress. It boosts NAD.

Some health-care clinics offer methylene blue in skin creams and intravenous infusions for people who want to improve memory and mood and slow down the aging process. Currently, the FDA has approved human use of methylene blue only for certain types of methemoglobinemia in which blood carries but does not release oxygen to cells. It is available on the retail market, but before trying it for longevity it's essential that you consult with a physician who is familiar with this drug, its dosage, and side effects. Too high a dose can cause toxicity. It is not unusual for your urine and skin to turn a shade of blue. The dose for longevity is unknown. Some people take 50 mg a day safely. There are concerns it can lead to gastric ulcer. It should not be taken by people with G6PD deficiency. Don't take methylene blue if you are taking a serotonin medication like an antidepressant because it can cause serotonin syndrome, which can be fatal.

Glutathione

Glutathione is one of the most promising life-extending molecules. It is one of the most abundant intracellular antioxidants in your system. This means it dramatically reduces the oxidative stress resulting from the imbalance between the production and degradation of reactive oxygen in cells. In other words, glutathione protects the cells. These by-products of normal oxygen metabolism accumulate in the body with age and interfere with chemical processes. Glutathione also improves brain function, mental clarity, and cognitive performance and shows promise in treating Parkinson's disease.

Unfortunately, as we age, glutathione, like other elements in the body, starts to decline, which contributes to inflammation and cell aging, which impairs cell communication. This speeds aging and can cause many diseases, including diabetes, arthritis, and cancer.

Glutathione is made up of three amino acids: glutamine, glycine, and cysteine. Researchers at Baylor College of Medicine in Houston, Texas, combined glycine and N-acetyl cysteine to create glyNAC to accelerate glutathione production. Their testing showed the positive effect of glutathione supplementation in mice that had reached their middle age of sixty-five weeks. Half the study mice were given glyNAC with food and lived 24 percent longer than those who ate untreated food. The second study showed positive results in mitochondrial function, nutrient sensing, and genomic stability, all factors in longevity.

Glutathione is available by injection (I take it as a shot whenever I have the chance), patches, and nasal sprays that target the central nervous system and the brain. It can be taken as a pill, but it is less effective in an oral form, although still worth taking. Glutathione is found in broccoli, parsley, garlic, spinach, Brussels sprouts, avocados, beets, and cabbage. Do whatever you need to boost your glutathione levels. The oral dose is 150–1500 mg a day.

Nattokinase

Are you concerned about a heart attack? Consider nattokinase. Nattokinase is an enzyme extracted and purified from a Japanese food called natto. Nattokinase prevents embolic blood clot formation and helps reduce blood pressure and reduces risk for stroke. In a twenty-six-week randomized study eighty-two volunteers who took 300 mg of nattokinase daily had the arterial wall and arterial plaques decreased by 36 percent. Don't take this supplement if you have had a hemorrhagic stroke, peptide ulcer, or coagulation disorder. Nattokinase dose is 100–300 mg a day.

Astaxanthin

Astaxanthin is one of the most powerful antioxidants on the planet. In fact, the Intervention Testing Program (ITP), a peer-reviewed program designed to identify agents that extended lifespan, confirmed its antioxidant activity against free radicals. This process cools inflammation, a hallmark of aging, and can be protective against cancer. This compound also helps keep our skin healthy and smooth as we get older. Research shows that astaxanthin extended the lifespan of mice by 12 percent, which translates into eight years in human life. Astaxanthin dose is 4–12 mg orally a day.

Supplements for Health and Beauty

These supplements not only play a role in beauty, but they also have anti-aging effects on your skin, joints, and overall health.

Collagen Peptides

As we age, we lose collagen from our skin. Collagen is like a rope that holds the skin together. By the time we are seventy, we lose 75 percent of all our collagen, which explains the wrinkles and saggy skin that occur as we grow older. Collagen peptides are destroyed by stomach acid, but hydrolyzed collagen peptides are absorbed more readily.

Research shows that people who take collagen peptides had better-looking skin than those who did not. Collagen peptides are safe. Supplementation also helps with joint pain, reduces inflammation in the joints, and slows age-related bone loss. It's safe to take up to 10 grams a day to have younger-looking skin as you age. I take this supplement in a gummy form. I also like to eat soups made with bone broth or choose bone marrow as an appetizer in restaurants.

Hyaluronic Acid

Want younger-looking skin? Hyaluronic acid is a sugar molecule found naturally in our bodies that declines as we age. Dermatologists inject hyaluronic acid as fillers in our faces, but you can also take it as a pill or in a face cream to promote younger-looking skin. It helps the skin retain moisture and even supports healthy joints. For radiant-looking skin, take 200 mg a day of hyaluronic acid a day.

Catalase

Hate your gray hair as you are getting older? Consider catalase. Catalase, an enzyme, is an alternative and natural approach to hair dyes. As we age, hydrogen peroxide, a natural by-product of metabolic reactions in the body, builds up in hair follicles and prevents the production of melanin that gives our hair color. Catalase converts hydrogen peroxide into stable, safe water and oxygen, but unfortunately, catalase decreases as we age. Load up on whole foods that are rich in zinc, copper, manganese, and selenium, which provide the body with the necessary components to make more catalase. All plants contain catalase, but there is more in kiwi, peaches, cherries, apricots, bananas, watermelon, and pineapple. Onions and garlic contain sulfur compounds that strengthen natural antioxidants like catalase and break down hydrogen peroxide. Vegetables that supply catalase include alfalfa, Brussels sprouts, cucumbers, parsnips, celery, red cabbage, leeks, radishes, kale, carrots, and spinach. Organically grown young sprouts of dark green plants are very high in catalase. According to the National Institutes of Health, sprouts like wheat and barley grass also contain catalase and antioxidants. Cooking decreases enzyme activity, so eat fruit and vegetables raw whenever you can. You can also buy catalase as a supplement and take 50 mg orally once a day.

Scientists are experimenting with hundreds of supplements to see their effects on the hallmarks of aging. We have very little human studies. I covered everything under the sun for you so you become a smart consumer. If you are feeling overwhelmed by the number of supplements in *The Ageless Revolution*, don't. They are not a must. I covered diet and exercise extensively; they are your first steps. Anything else is extra. Some biohackers take fifty supplements or more and are able to reverse their biological age by fifteen years or more, but you don't need to follow in their footsteps.

Decide on which supplements to take based on your own needs. For example, if you live in a cloudy area, with no sun, take vitamin D3. If you have concerns about heart attacks, consider nattokinase.

Keep in mind if you eat right and exercise, you do not need to take any supplements. However, depleted soils make most fruits and vegetables less nutritious, so a supplement can help fill in this gap. I think of supplements as insurance. Also, none of us are perfect. It's nearly impossible to eat perfectly 24-7. Most of us can't forage for our meals, eat all organic foods, or live in Blue Zones. Supplements can help us survive and thrive despite the modern lifestyle assault on our cells and body.

Supplements: Why They're Worth It

Personally, I take twenty to twenty-five-plus pills a day and add more as new research shows benefits for longevity. Many of the supplements I take are spices such as saffron, Ceylon cinnamon, or from that list. I attempt to do it on most days. This runs me $200–$300 a month. I know this could be costly, but I tried my very best to make it affordable for everyone. For sure, I am on the extreme as I got educated. I think taking four to five supplements that are based on human studies is quite enough. If you decide to go further based on animal studies, it would be your choice.

For the price of a few well-chosen supplements, a fraction of what I recommend, you may be able to fully live your life in good health for another ten or twenty years! You can also continue to earn income during this time for your later years. Not to mention the money you'll save on medications and medical care. Think of the time you will spend with your friends and family, pursuing new dreams, hobbies, and giving back to the community and the world. Priceless.

You can make room in your budget for several important supplements. You just need to reevaluate your priorities. You may decide to cut back on eating out or ordering in, trim your cable bill, or skip a few lattes.

Which Supplements Should You Take First?

If I had to choose from this huge list, I would recommend that you take fish oil, taurine, NR, vitamin D3, selenium, ubiquinol, astaxanthin, and low-dose vitamin K2 daily. This should not cost more than $120–$130 a month. It all depends on your age, too, and where you live. I have partnered with *Life Extension* magazine to give readers of *The Ageless Revolution* huge discounts and make it easy for them to get high-quality supplements from a reputable high-quality brand. I want an affordable revolution. You will find their toll-free number in the Appendix. No promises if you decide to be a guinea pig like those animals who took the supplements and lived longer.

Start with three to five supplements. In time, you can add more as you continue your ageless journey. Follow label directions as to when to take each supplement and whether to take it with food or not. You'll find more information about each supplement on the book website: www.TheAgelessRevolution.com.

Remember . . .

The list of the supplements discussed in this chapter are suggestions, they are not a must in *The Ageless Revolution*. Be sure to consult with your doctor before trying any of them. If you take any, start slowly, with three or four supplements. Later add more.

- Fish oil 1 gram a day.
- Taurine 1,500–3,000 mg a day.
- Fisetin 500 mg a day.
- Resveratrol 1 gram of trans-resveratrol daily or less. It can be harmful at high doses.
- Pterostilbene 150 mg a day.
- Quercetin 500–1,000 mg a day.
- NR 300 mg daily.
- NMN 1 gram a day.
- Trimethyglycine (TMG) 1 gram a day.
- Vitamin D3 5,000–10,000 IU a day with natural fats such as yogurt or some nuts.
- Astragalus Root 100–500 IU a day.
- Plasmalogens 0.5 mg a day if no brain disease.
- Vitamin K2 45 mcg a day.
- Carnosine 500–2,000 mg a day.
- Glucosamine 1,500 mg a day.
- Calcium alpha-ketoglutarate 1–2 grams a day.
- Catalase 50 mg a day.

- Selenium 100–200 mcg a day.
- Ubiquinol 100–200 mg a day.
- Nattokinase 100–300 mg a day.
- Astaxanthin 4–12 mg a day.
- Collagen peptides 10 grams a day.
- Hyaluronic acid 200 mg a day.

CHAPTER 17

Get More Good Stress

What doesn't kill you makes you stronger!
—Kelly Clarkson

Stress sucks up your energy, negatively affects your brain, and shortens your telomeres. I shared with you earlier my very personal story of how stress nearly killed me with both depression and suicidal thoughts when I didn't even realize that I was stressed.

But there is a good type of stress for our cells to make us stronger; it is called hormesis.

A Different Type of Stress Is Actually Good for You

Stress is disruption of homeostasis, or your body's status of equilibrium. When you exercise, you damage your muscles, so you build new muscle fibers. When you learn a different language, you build new connections between your brain cells. When you get a laser treatment on your face at your dermatologist, you damage your skin, and stimulate the growth of new skin and collagen.

Both exercise and intermittent fasting are forms of hormesis. Even alcohol in small doses has a hormetic effect because it damages your mitochondria and causes inflammation of your gut. One thing for sure: I do not advocate alcohol as a hormetic stressor.

Have a Good Stressful Day at the Spa

When most people go to the spa, they think of a day of relaxation, and getting a professional massage or a facial. But if you want to live longer, a different spa experience is needed. Instead, I encourage you to experience extreme cold and hot temperatures to activate your sirtuins, the emergency repair genes for your cells. You already activated your sirtuins on *The Ageless Revolution* by eating clean and exercising, but let us take it up a notch.

Taking Stress to the Next Level

If you want to live a longer, fully healthier life, with increased physical performance and an optimized mental state, it's necessary to think outside the normal spa experience.

Adversity is the key to longevity. Sirtuins, the longevity proteins and the CEO of our cells, switch off when we are comfortable. They switch on in stressful situations. Extreme cold switches sirtuins on, and when they are activated, you become biologically stronger after the experience. Keep in mind that adversity was part of early human life. Extreme temperatures were the norm. There were no heaters or air conditioners. That is why, despite my definite preference for a relaxed day at the spa getting a massage, I became super fascinated by super-cold treatment chambers. Freezing for longevity has physiology, psychology, and science behind it.

Cryotherapy

The use of extreme cold as a medical treatment has been around for a long time. People apply ice to provide pain relief for inflamed, injured, or overused muscles. Pro athletes soak a sore limb, or their entire body, in a tub of ice water; that is called cold water immersion (CWI).

Cold-stress therapy and its new, popular poster child, whole-body cryotherapy (WBC), have recently gained popularity with athletes. Both techniques work with the phenomenon of hormesis, whereby the body reaps certain benefits when it is exposed to low doses of a stressor—in this case, cold. Doctors and scientists do not yet fully understand all the potential benefits and risks of this process. But, that said, cold-stress therapy, along with its opposite treatment, heat-stress therapy, are increasingly credited with a wide range of positive physical and mental benefits, some of which are supported by international scientific studies.

In the health spa setting, whole-body cryotherapy means standing almost naked. You must wear heavy socks, gloves, a headband or beanie, and a mask (to protect your airways) in an enclosed cryotherapy chamber. Some cryotherapy uses nitrogen for the cold temperature to be produced, so you only immerse your body and not your face.

The temperature surrounding your body in the cryosauna is −175°F. You might be saying, "Doc, I would rather die than step into a chamber at −175°F!" But this treatment only takes from two minutes forty-five seconds to three minutes fifteen seconds. Again, nothing in my book is my personal opinion.

You decide how much you can tolerate. The attendant can adjust your cold level endurance with a fan on a scale from one to five, and of course, you have the option to get out at any time.

Cryotherapy is indeed super cold, but people find whole-body cryotherapy to be surprisingly bearable and—placebo effect or not—invigorating. I am sure if you live in a cold city, you have seen a polar plunge in an ocean near you. They do it in the Scandinavian countries all the time. And, let us face it, it is hard to say no to the idea of unlocking the power within our own bodies to help us enjoy happier, healthier, and stronger lives.

Extreme cold can be a challenge to endure, but it can give you focus. It can encourage you to stay on track with other aspects of your longevity program.

After investing time, energy, and courage into conquering cryotherapy, I doubt you will want to eat a piece of candy or put a cookie in your mouth again and undo the health progress you have accomplished. You are activating your sirtuins, one of the pathways in nutrient sensing. You certainly would not be motivated to impair your IGF-1 and AMPK pathways with a cookie! Or impairing your sirtuins with bacon from the newest low-carb diet on the market. Cryotherapy promises a list of benefits, including pain relief and muscle healing, improved post-injury rehabilitation, improved athletic performance, reduced inflammation, prevention and treatment of chronic diseases, prevention of dementia, boosting the immune system, and reducing anxiety and depression.

The Iceman Cometh

Wim Hof, "The Iceman," is a Dutch motivational speaker. He brought attention to cryotherapy to the public. He earned his nickname and global fame with twenty-six Guinness World Records for exposure to extreme cold and heat—including climbing to 22,000 feet on Mount Everest wearing nothing but shorts and shoes and running a marathon in the 120-degree Saharan desert heat without water. Do not challenge his record. Following the sudden death of his wife in 1995, Hof used his understanding of nature and extreme cold to heal himself of the emotional trauma he suffered. Now, his personal bio-experimentation is taking him, and us all, into fascinating and groundbreaking territory. In the beautiful, unforgiving laboratory of nature, Hof uses tummo-like breathing with visualization during his exposure to extreme cold. Tummo breathing is an ancient breathing technique that increases a person's internal heat.

Practice Tummo Breathing

If you decide to try cryotherapy, tummo breathing is often done with it. Tummo breathing, which translates into inner fire, is an ancient breathwork technique originally practiced by the Tibetan Buddhist monks. I find myself doing it unintentionally when I enter a cryotherapy chamber. Wim Hof's method and tummo breathing are remarkably similar. Breathing raises the body temperature. You relax, clear your mind, and visualize a fire around your belly button.

Once you're in the chamber, place your hands around your stomach, curl your spine, and exhale strongly with rounded lips as if you are blowing through a straw. Breathe in and out five times. As you do, inhale, hold the inhale, and push the air out with your diaphragm and pelvic floors. Repeat the sequence. You'll notice the heat starts to build in your belly. This is a good breathing technique to do when you are freezing!

Is Cryotherapy Right for You?

Hof trains people to connect with and influence their own autonomic nervous systems. He aims to empower people to work with their own bodies' adrenal and immune systems to fight various devastating autoimmune diseases and the related, debilitating issues of depression, fear, anxiety, and pain.

Hof's dedication to his work is amazing, and the results are stunning. Thousands of testimonials from people around the world speak to the global reach of, and interest in, Hof's message. Researchers around the world at major universities are currently exploring the underlying medical science and potential of Hof's work.

There is considerable speculation that the meditative elements and personal challenges that are central to Wim Hof's approach are important contributors to the positive impact people have experienced.

Is Cryotherapy Safe for You to Try?

Be sure to consult with a physician to determine if cryotherapy is safe for you. Dr. Robert H. Shmerling, a faculty editor of *Harvard Health Publishing*, states:

> While whole body cryotherapy is considered safe and few problems have been reported with its use, some people are advised to avoid WBC because it may worsen conditions such as:
> - Poorly controlled high blood pressure
> - Major heart or lung disease
> - Poor circulation such as Raynaud's disease (it gets much

worse with exposure to cold)
- Allergy symptoms triggered by cold
- Neuropathy (nerve disease) in the legs or feet.

You can find a cryotherapy spa in your city; do it once or twice a week if you can. Typically, I go once or twice a month. Not inexpensive, the session typically costs fifty to sixty-five dollars. (No worries, I will offer affordable alternatives.) If you have no underlying health issues, it is quite safe. Some spas have monthly memberships just like gym memberships.

How Does Cryotherapy Keep Us Young?

We have no longevity studies on cryotherapy, but it appears to have numerous anti-aging effects. So how does cryotherapy affect anti-aging? There are several mechanisms. We have three types of fats in our bodies: white fat, brown fat, and beige fat. Brown fat, mostly located between our scapula or shoulder blades, is good. This type of fat regulates body temperature, burns calories, and stores energy. It secretes youth factors.

White fat is bad. It's found around our bellies, and it comes from excess calories. White fat secretes inflammatory chemicals that promote aging.

Beige fat is a mixture of white and brown fat. Babies have lots of brown fat. We lose brown fat as we age, and we tend to gain more white fat. Cryotherapy helps you build brown fat, meaning more youth factors circulating in your blood. It's thought that cryotherapy also helps build collagen in the skin. Who wouldn't love that?

I found that I was able to endure more time in the cold chamber and build more tolerance as I did more sessions. I take off my clothes, protect my ears and fingers, and ask the attendant for three minutes and fifteen seconds while working on my breathing. I get some music going, the time passes quickly, and I come out feeling rejuvenated. I try to have a positive attitude since I am doing unimaginable things.

To make *The Ageless Revolution* affordable, as an alternative for those who find cryotherapy cost prohibitive, try taking a very cold bath once a week.

Start by filling the tub with water, then drop in two to three buckets of ice. Stay in the tub for seven to ten minutes. You'll feel refreshed afterward, and your skin will look better. Or find a gym with a cold plunge pool. If you live close to an ocean or lake, take a cold polar plunge in the winter. You can also always set your thermostat at 65°F. Or take a walk in the winter. Exposure to cold in all its forms can stimulate production of brown fat and help build collagen. At the present time, we don't have any information if cryotherapy can help with human longevity.

The Benefits of Infrared Sauna Treatment

Do you prefer not to be frozen? Then go for the heat. In Finland, saunas are a way of life. It is where business deals are sealed and friendships forged. Heat may do the same activation for your sirtuins proteins. Again, your sirtuins alert your cells that there is a danger ahead. It is a surviving trigger. Infrared sauna treatment can provide you with most of the same benefits as freezing your bottom off, as well as offering some new ones. Sauna sessions promote circulation, cleanse the pores, and leave you feeling rejuvenated. Infrared sauna is also an excellent way to get rid of the toxins we piled up in our fat. Extreme heat might remind you of a vacation in the Amazon jungle, or the last time your air-conditioning went out in midsummer.

Infrared sauna therapy stimulates your mitochondria to produce adenosine triphosphate (ATP). When the mitochondria are healthy, you will feel more energetic. You will also be less likely to suffer from the risk of heart disease or cancer. That is because you increase blood flow to your organs and increase your heat tolerance, strength, and endurance. Furthermore, your heart benefits because heat can reduce high blood pressure by expanding the blood vessels and reducing the thickening of the carotid arteries. Studies done on Finnish men who use the hot sauna regularly revealed they had less cardiovascular disease and heart attacks than men who did not use the sauna. This type of sauna can also restore cell function, decrease vascular inflammation, and improve cellular strength, therefore building resistance to stress.

In Alzheimer's disease, damaged protein cells cluster in the brain, which leads to cell death. Heat therapy can often reverse the initial cell damage and promote regrowth in them. It also keeps neurons healthy by increasing how fast the neurons regenerate and grow.

Using infrared sauna treatment increases stem cell survival and function. Stem cells can move more quickly through the affected tissue to lessen pain and enhance healing. Speaking of pain, heat therapy is also helpful for pain management. With the increased blood flow that treatment brings, more oxygen and nutrients are absorbed by the cells of the body. Increased oxygen helps to relax muscle pain and relieve joint and arthritic pain.

As your core temperature rises in the sauna, your body produces white blood cells as it would if you had a fever. Your body can fight illness with more white blood cells, rallying to the call for help. Although infrared saunas should not be used for weight loss, the rise of internal body temperature does increase your metabolism. Some claim that an infrared sauna session can burn up to 600 calories in one hour. Of course, a hot sauna should not be your way of burning calories.

If you are prescribed heat for detoxification, sweating in the sauna will also help your blood flow to important organs while purging toxins and impurities like heavy metals, nicotine, and certain industrial compounds like phthalates. Phthalates are nasty salts that disrupt hormones. They have been linked to breast cancer, low sperm count in men, early puberty, infertility, and birth defects.

Infrared sauna can also purge traces of drugs like LSD, which are stored in fatty tissues. It may have been years since you used drugs, but even so, the drug is released little by little into the rest of your body. Sometimes it is not noticed, but sometimes it can cause physical and mental cravings for the drug, and even full-blown flashbacks.

There can also be a residue of antidepressants, sedatives, chemotherapy, anesthetics, and other medications that are still in fat cells. Chances are, however, that your body will quickly detoxify these. If prescribed heat therapy, be sure to tell your doctor about any past drug use—legal or otherwise—and have someone supervise you in the sauna.

There are some risks, including heat exhaustion and dehydration. Be sure to drink plenty of water before, during, and after your sauna session. While in the sauna, do not pour water on yourself. Let your body temperature go up.

After the sauna, continue to drink some water every fifteen minutes for an hour. Some medicine can be affected by the intense sauna heat, increased blood circulation, and sweating.

Insulin and transdermal patches can make using the sauna dangerous. Ask your doctor about any medications you're taking and potential problems with heat therapy interacting with the medicines you are taking. For example, people suffering from certain medical conditions should not use infrared sauna treatment.

Among the risks are heart attack, aortic stenosis, stroke caused by brain bleed, unstable angina pectoris, lupus, brain tumors, and multiple sclerosis. People with diabetes, pacemakers, and titanium implants for bones and joints need to be cautious and discuss heat treatment with their doctor before getting into a sauna. Wow, that sounds like the disclaimers for drugs advertised on television! Preferably, ask your physician because that is the person who should know your medical history best. Overall, infrared sauna treatment is safe when prescribed by your doctor or licensed practitioner, assuming you have discussed all health issues and medicines you are taking with them. If you do not have the money to go to sessions at your local spa, there are several at-home sauna alternatives that provide similar benefits.

You can invest in a portable sauna; it is a space saver. You can fold it after you are done and store it anywhere. You can also buy a sauna blanket. It is about a hundred dollars. It is certainly more affordable than an infrared sauna that costs thousands of dollars. You get in it after wearing some cotton clothes as it gets hot on your skin. You are not totally in; your head will be out. You sweat for one hour. If you do not want to bother buying a sauna or a portable sauna at all, no worries! Although not as beneficial as an infrared sauna, a steam shower at your local gym will do too. So go to your local gym and use their sauna. Steam sauna provides the heat, but not the infrared benefits.

Hormetic stress has its place in anti-aging. The research shows us the benefits of such measures. It is a new era to age. No excuses. I have given you lots of affordable measures if these procedures are cost prohibitive. Get those sirtuins fired up.

Remember . . .

- *Cryotherapy* is a challenge but find a spa or gym that offers it. Or just use your own bathtub! Run the cold water, add plenty of ice, and get in. While you are in there, practice staying longer, up to ten minutes.

- *Tummo* breathing is a form of meditation breathing that can teach you to rev your internal furnace to keep you warm during a cryo-therapy session. Check it out online.

- *Infrared sauna treatments* make you sweat more than a regular sauna, but the benefits are far greater. They help you get rid of toxins. You can find them in spas, gyms, and free-standing facil-ities. If you cannot find an infrared, use your regular gym sauna a few times a week. Drink lots of water before, during, and after your sauna. If you can afford it, buy an infrared blanket for home use.

PART V

Taking *The Ageless Revolution* to the Next Level with Professional Help

CHAPTER 18

Turn Back Time

We know what we are but know not what we may be.
—**William Shakespeare**

Cells need to communicate. *The Ageless Revolution* will help you balance insulin, which is related to excess sugar intake. It will help balance leptin, which is disturbed by trans fats. It will boost your growth hormone with exercise. It will help lower your cortisol, the stress hormone, as you meditate. But what about the vanishing sex hormones?

Many anti-aging books discuss metformin, intermittent fasting, and that's where the conversation ends! Not good. We also need our sex hormones as we get older. We need to target all the hallmarks of aging, not just one or two!

For this reason, I feel that the time has come for all doctors to treat the hormonal imbalance that we all face as we get old. If you decide to go any further in your anti-aging journey, you will need to find the right medical professional or professionals who can help you with those measures.

No celebrity has shed the spotlight on bioidentical hormones and sex hormones more than Suzanne Somers. I met Suzanne in 2010 for the first time at a medical conference in Las Vegas. I was always impressed by her passion to bring anti-aging information to the masses. Throughout the years, many editors of magazines and newspapers asked me to comment on her books, so I familiarized myself with her work.

When I met Suzanne again a few years later, I apologized to her because I'd been misquoted as attacking her views in an article in a major newspaper when I really agreed with what she said. After all, much of her information came from my colleagues and doctors with whom I speak or work. The editor for the newspaper was in a rush for the article and never gave me the chance to proofread it. It was truly my mistake.

She didn't seem annoyed but firmly replied, "I am always attacked for my views." During the height of the pandemic, we were in a Zoom meeting, and she talked enthusiastically about her favorite subject—hormones. When I heard of Suzanne's death, I was in shock and felt very sad. She was a true pioneer in anti-aging.

For a moment, I wondered whether I should even challenge death in *The Ageless Revolution* in its final stages. I told a very good friend of mine that maybe *The Ageless Revolution* should be about healthy living. We truly have no say, no matter what we do, to control our fate. My friend told me something very inspirational: "Michael, never lose sight of your new direction. You are on to something big that was never done before; you should be an inspiration and a beacon of hope for all people." He was totally right. I was derailed momentarily by Suzanne's death. There are certainly no guarantees in life, but we must do our very best to live healthier. Hopefully, if we are lucky, those positive measures will make us live a very long life. And this brings me to this chapter to discuss hormones.

Aging and the Loss of Sex Hormones

Cells need to talk with one another, and one way they do that is by hormones. This is vitally important because impaired cell communication is one of the ten hallmarks of aging. Some hormones build muscles, bones, and tissues, others like insulin regulate blood sugar. As we age, one of the biggest issues we face is the loss of our sex hormones, which include estrogen, progesterone, and testosterone. Suzanne Somers was passionate about this topic and wrote several books, including one published in 2007, called *Ageless*, especially dedicated to hormones.

Sex hormones need to be replaced as we get older. You can drink all the black tea you want, eat all the sweet purple potatoes you want, but that's not enough to turn back time by thirty, forty, or fifty years when sex organs shut down. You need to do more, much more. You need your sex hormones replaced to feel alive.

Women live almost half their adult life in nonreproductive years and often suffer from low energy, fatigue, poor sleep, and a low libido. One in every four men in America has low testosterone. Fatigue, loss of muscle mass, and low libido is what men experience.

Bioidentical Hormone Replacement

The good news, with bioidentical hormone replacement, sixty or even seventy is now the new twenty. You read that right. It's all about hormone replacement as we get older.

Yes, aging is a fact of life. But you've seen that there are many ways, through diet and lifestyle, to renew your youthful vitality and appearance, improve your health, and ward off illness through eating clean, exercising, and intermittent fasting. You can make your cells young again. Bioidentical hormones are one way to do that.

See Your Health-Care Practitioner About Natural Hormone Replacement

So how can you get your youth back when your sex hormones vanish? If you are a woman in menopause or a man diagnosed with low testosterone, it is time to find a doctor who can help you with natural hormone replacement. Hormones get a bad rap in the media as usually synthetic hormones are confused with natural hormones. If you have low sex hormones, you need to replace them. You can see an experienced primary care doctor, your gynecologist if you are female, or your urologist if you are male.

When Do You Need Sex Hormones?

Of course, if you are in your twenties or thirties and reading this book, you don't need to worry about hormone replacement unless you have a problem. For women, you do not need to worry about hormone replacement unless you are in menopause, perimenopause, had your ovaries removed, or are experiencing irregular periods.

Andropause is the male equivalent of menopause in women. Testosterone starts to decline in men starting from age twenty-five! Gentlemen, consult a doctor if you suspect you have low testosterone and you have symptoms such as low sex drive, erectile dysfunction, fatigue, weight gain, and low energy. At age fifty, most men are already in andropause.

Menopause

During female menopause, the ovaries shut down. Estrogen and pro-gesterone decline precipitously. Uncomfortable symptoms, like hot flashes, night sweats, headaches, vaginal dryness, mental fuzziness, frequent bladder infections, weight gain, and decreased sexual drive, occur. This dual hormone drop increases a woman's risk for osteoporosis, heart disease, and cancer. It feels like nature is telling us, "It is over, your youth and vitality are gone, time to go."

Estrogen and progesterone are both produced primarily in the ovaries, but a small amount is also produced in the adrenal glands. In women, these hormone levels vary in relation to ovulation.

Estrogen gives women their curvy appearance, lowers body fat, protects against heart disease and Alzheimer's disease, and increases insulin sensi-tivity. During reproductive years, a woman naturally makes estrogen every day of the month. When estrogen production stops, symptoms of that hor-mone deficiency can happen at any age, but they are more prominent in menopause. Estrogen is uniquely three different types of hormones: estrone, estradiol, and estriol.

Three Types of Estrogen

1. Estrone
2. Estradiol
3. Estriol

Estrone is made mostly in the fat and mainly after menopause. Estradiol is made in the ovaries; it is the main estrogen made in the reproductive years. Estriol is also made in the ovaries; it is only made during pregnancy.

But estrogen is not the only female sex hormone that goes down in menopause. Estrogen is counteracted by another hormone, progesterone, which is also produced by the ovaries. Progesterone reduces anxiety and has a calming effect on mood, preventing depression. During a woman's reproductive years, progesterone is secreted for two weeks each month. It coincides with the ovulation part of the menstrual cycle. A lack of progesterone can happen at any time, not just in menopause.

Postpartum depression happens with the precipitous drop of progesterone after the birth of a baby. This form of depression should be treated with progesterone replacement rather than with antidepressants. Progesterone improves sleep, helps support bones, helps mature breast tissue, and prepares breasts to produce milk.

Progesterone protects women against breast cancer. Have you noticed that breast cancer happens more often in women right during or after menopause? Estradiol, which is the main hormone produced in reproductive years, vanishes, and a woman is left with estrone, the type of estrogen that promotes cancer. Progesterone, which opposes estrogen, vanishes, and the risk of cancer goes up.

Low progesterone levels can happen at any age, but production usually plummets around menopause. Symptoms of progesterone deficiency include PMS-like symptoms, premenstrual migraines, irregular and heavy periods, depression, and anxiety.

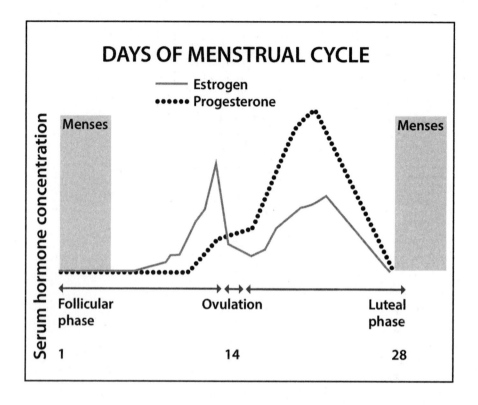

My Mother's Journey Through Menopause

Growing up, I remember my poor mother who went through menopause at age fifty in one of the worst ways possible. When my mom's periods
stopped, she would lose her temper and would scream at me and my sister
at the top of her lungs for seemingly no reason. She also cried inconsolably
all the time for no reason. She alternated between feeling hot and cold and
sweated profusely all the time.

As a child, I thought she had lost her mind. But she had no family history
of mental issues. For more than two years, she continued to suffer. No doctor
was able to help her. They all told her, "Your hormones are normal!" Often
my patients tell me that they have been told the same thing by their gynecol-
ogists. Yes, hormones might be normal for your age when you are in menopause, but this doesn't mean that women have enough of these hormones

(the way they did when they were in their twenties) to feel good. You can't compare your levels to someone your age. You should compare yourself to the young person you can be.

Often doctors treat those menopausal symptoms with antidepressants, tranquilizers, or synthetic hormones. This is no fix!

Synthetic hormones are in fact made from pregnant horses' urine and sold as pharmaceuticals with names such as Premarin and Prempro. With them comes the risk of blood clots, stroke, heart disease, breast cancer, damaged arteries, and death. We are humans, not horses.

Yes, you will feel better temporarily with those drugs, but these synthetic hormones will shorten your life. It is so sad to see that we are brainwashed to eat cereals made with refined carbs and low-fat products with added chemicals that make us sick; encouraged to eat fake fats like margarine; and when women reach menopause, they are treated with sex hormones from horses! Sadly, doctors too often do not challenge conventional allopathic medicine dictums that often do more harm than good. This is thanks to billionaires including the Rockefellers, Vanderbilts, and the Carnegies who nearly stamped out holistic or alternative medicines in the early twentieth century. Medicine is mostly today about treating the symptoms rather than dealing with the root cause of disease.

Today, natural remedies are rarely taught in medical schools or residency training programs. This is because these institutions receive grants from pharmaceutical companies that sell standard, patented drugs. I used to be one of those doctors, following the herd; I never questioned the authorities until one day, I woke up. I used my brain and trusted myself more than these prestigious institutions who tell us to eat fake foods. I couldn't follow the same path. I also have a voice that I can use to educate people. I became aware of how many of the medicines that are commonly prescribed aren't helpful and can be harmful, including synthetic hormones.

In fact, in 2002, the Women's Health Initiative study trial alerted doctors to the danger of synthetic hormones that had been used for decades. As

I've said, these synthetic hormones increase women's risk for heart attacks, stroke, breast cancer, and early death. As a result, there was an increased interest in the use of bioidentical hormones after Suzanne Somers became a strong advocate for them.

What Are Bioidentical Hormones?

Bioidentical hormones have the same makeup as those sex hormones naturally produced in your body. They are derived from a molecule called diosgenin, found in yam and soy. Bioidentical hormones are quite different from the synthetic hormone replacement drugs given by most doctors.

You can get those natural sex hormones from compounding pharmacies or your local pharmacy. Compounded bioidentical hormone replacement therapy (CBHRT) uses combined bioidentical hormones in a personalized, made-to-order prescription. It is not a cookie-cutter hormone.

The FDA, which does not prohibit the compounding of bioidentical hormones, has approved several formulations of bioidentical estradiol and progesterone that are molecularly identical to the structure of the hormones generated by the human body. However, the FDA doesn't approve any specific compounded products, for any condition, because the products are not standardized.

Are Compounded Bioidentical Hormones Safe?

In a word, yes, if you use a reputable pharmacy. Compounding pharmacists from reputable pharmacies have been preparing medications with an excellent record for safety and effectiveness prior to the advent of mass-produced pharmaceuticals. There is strict regulation and oversight of compounding bioidentical hormones.

I have used bioidentical hormones in my practice for years, long before the FDA approved many of these natural hormones as patented drugs obtainable from regular pharmacies.

Compounding pharmacies are regulated by each state's pharmacy board and the Pharmaceutical Compounding Accreditation Board. Each state's regulations require consistency in purity and dosage. There is a regulation by the U.S. Pharmacopeia and the Code of Federal Regulations, which requires purity testing.

The prescriptions filled out at compounding pharmacies have hormones that are FDA approved and are obtained from FDA-inspected and -approved facilities. And compounded hormones do not need FDA approval since they are not mass-produced.

How to Start on Bioidentical Hormones

You will need to see a doctor who is experienced in bioidentical hormone replacement. You can get a script from him or her and go to your local compounding pharmacy or regular pharmacy depending on what the doctor ordered. Women need estrogen and progesterone when they are in perimenopause and menopause and sometimes, an exceptionally low dose of testosterone to get their libido back. Bioidentical hormones and compounded bioidentical hormones can be delivered in various ways. Sustained release of estrogen that comes as a patch or pellet may be more effective for severe vasomotor symptoms. A pellet is like a reservoir placed by your doctor under the skin to deliver small amounts of estrogen. It is placed every few months.

Bioidentical hormones also come in other forms including gels, sublingual pills, and vaginal creams. These formulations expose the body to a smaller dose of natural estrogen every day. Progesterone, which helps with sleep, should be taken two weeks a month rather than continuously to mimic a young woman's ovulation cycles.

Progesterone can be taken daily, but it may lead to weight gain. I am adamantly opposed to daily progesterone since nature intended for women to make progesterone for two weeks only each month. If you are a woman in menopause, consult with your doctor, but ask him or her to use only bioidentical hormones.

Pharmaceutical or Bioidentical Hormones: Which Are Better and Why?

Now that the FDA allows natural hormones as drugs, you don't have to use compounding pharmacies. Your doctor can prescribe natural hormones that are standardized, FDA approved, and dispensed by major pharmaceutical companies. They are covered by insurance. Estrogen is available in major pharmacy chains under brand names that include Vivelle-Dot (generic), Climara, Estradiol, and others. You can attach one of those patches with a small dose of estrogen in it to your skin once a week or insert a small amount of cream in your vagina once a day.

Estrogen should not be taken orally or in pill form because it increases a woman's risk for stroke. It must be counteracted with progesterone in cream or oral form, which is safe. This oral progesterone is sold under the name Prometrium.

Make sure the progesterone you take is natural. Do not confuse bioidentical progesterone with progesterone that is synthetic. The labels should say progesterone, not medroxyprogesterone or any other ingredient with too many syllables!

When Is Testosterone Needed for Women?

Testosterone, the male sex hormone, is also needed in women, but in very small amounts. It is also lost with age. Sometimes, a woman may need a little natural testosterone to get her libido back. Without sufficient testosterone, a woman can experience mood swings, depression, low libido, lack of focus, reduced strength, and loss of lean body mass. A prescription for an exceptionally low dose of testosterone cream could be all that is needed to adjust for the testosterone deficiency. So a compounding pharmacy will be needed. Unbelievably, there is not a single testosterone hormone drug on the market that is manufactured by drug companies for women. For Big Pharma, it is like women in menopause were never meant to have a sex drive! An experienced doctor can guide with the right dose.

Advice About Taking Bioidentical or Pharmaceutical Natural Hormones

Regardless of what you get, compounded or pharmaceutical natural hormones, start on a low dose and increase the dose gradually if menopause symptoms are still present. Remember, the goal in menopause is not fertility but health and longevity. I often suggest using an estrogen patch of 0.5 mg once a week and some progesterone as cream or a pill two weeks of each month at a dose of 100 mg a day. Again, a little bit of testosterone cream daily may also be needed from a compounding pharmacy. Make sure to have a mammogram with normal results before starting sex hormones and have no family history of breast or ovarian cancer. You may be in menopause, but you are like twenty again. The good news, those bioidentical hormones have been linked to longevity.

For Men: Andropause or Low Testosterone

With all the toxins around us, testosterone levels in men are declining at rapid speed even in the younger generation in the United States. Andropause is the male equivalent of female menopause. Low testosterone is happening now in every age group. Normal lab levels are 241–827 ng/dL, but levels plummet as men age.

For years, the medical community has told the public that testosterone supplementation leads to prostate cancer. That is simply not true. Testosterone replacement therapy has no link to prostate cancer whatsoever.

Testosterone: A Total Body Hormone for Men

Testosterone hormone is produced in the testes and is the essence of being a man. It makes men masculine. It improves libido. But testosterone is not just a sex hormone—it is a total body hormone. In adult males, testosterone is necessary to keep muscle mass and strength, bone mass, normal hair growth, libido, and sperm production. It also keeps men fit and lean. Unfortunately, athletes who abuse steroids have given testosterone a bad reputation.

Testosterone is mostly bound to a protein, called serum hormone binding globulin, so all the action of testosterone really comes from a small fraction, which is the free testosterone. I often explain to my patients free testosterone by this analogy: Imagine having a house, which is your net worth (total testosterone), and the cash in the bank is the money available to function (free testosterone). So if you have a $500,000 house, which is your total testosterone, but don't have any money in the bank, you can't feel good because you are money poor. All the action of testosterone is coming from the free testosterone, not the bound testosterone. So it is important to look at the levels of free testosterone as well.

The Problem with Lab Tests for Testosterone

When you get assessed for testosterone levels, the lab will often show you what is considered the "normal" range among patients who have tested at that lab. It is called the "reference range." Here is the problem: the reference range consists of a *wide* variety of men who tested with that specific lab: eighty-year-old men and twenty-year-old men; obese men and super fit men; men with a pituitary gland problem and men with a normal gland.

For example, Quest lab shows a reference range of 300–800 ng/dl (nanograms per deciliter) for total testosterone levels. According to this reference range, a twenty-year-old with a level of total testosterone of 300 ng/dl will fall within the normal range, when in fact, his levels are exceptionally low for his age.

The fact that reference ranges do not break patients down by age or health status explains why a twenty-five-year-old man can go to his doctor with the symptoms of low testosterone, only to be told that his levels are fine because they are within the "normal" lab's range. His levels are normal only based on the lab because he is compared to an eighty-year-old man. His diagnosis of low testosterone is missed! I certainly don't want to have the testosterone level of an eighty-year-old man, and you should not too. Guidelines should be adjusted based on each patient's age.

Why Do Testosterone Levels Decline?

I told you age-related diseases are happening now much more in younger people. Testosterone levels are declining in men across America from toxins and processed food. It is a disaster. Although eating a healthy diet can improve longevity, lifestyle choices and other factors can also influence hormonal imbalance. This accelerates the aging process at the cellular level and can set you on the path toward disease. Other factors that cause testosterone hormone to deplete are aging, obesity, stress, illness, smoking, drugs and alcohol use, depression, fake fats, mental illness, and not enough sexual activity.

The symptoms of testosterone deficiency are baldness, reduced body hair, less muscle, more fat accumulation, and reduced strength and stamina. Because testosterone decreases so slowly, over decades, many men think the subtle symptoms of andropause are just part of the normal aging process. We are told to accept it!

Sexual symptoms of a problem are decreased sex drive, reduced organ sensitivity or pleasure, fewer orgasms, and erectile dysfunction. Some medical professionals may tell us "Live with it! Accept your age! I will give you a script for Viagra!" But there is more that can be done that's good for you.

Problems Caused by Declining Testosterone

The danger of declining testosterone does not stop here. Cardiovascular problems are increased by more abdominal fat bringing a greater risk of heart attack; higher insulin, cholesterol, and triglyceride levels; and high blood pressure. Mental issues happen such as moodiness, irritability, anxiety, poor concentration, memory loss, and less efficient critical thinking. All these issues are often treated with psychiatric medications. Again, this is no fix.

Current medical research also shows that low testosterone levels may be associated with benign prostatic hyperplasia (BPH), or an enlarged prostate. This is because the prostate gland goes through a second growth spurt as men reach their forties, fifties, and sixties, and this can result in benign prostatic hyperplasia (BPH).

As the prostate grows, it pushes on the bladder and urethra, causing mild to severe urinary discomforts such as increased frequency of urination, especially at night, difficulty starting urination, decreased urinary force, and the sensation of a full bladder, even after urinating.

This happens because as the body senses declining testosterone with age it compensates by producing a form of super testosterone called dihydrotestosterone, and this leads to an enlarged prostate.

At the same time, estrogen levels still are the same or increase as men gain weight around their bellies. This elevated estrogen hormone level leads to signs of aging such as enlargement of male breasts and less body hair.

Testosterone Replacement Therapy

The earlier that a testosterone imbalance is detected and treated, the better. Testosterone replacement therapy (TRT) supplements can give you symptom relief while delaying other age-related declines. But you have to address your diet, sleep, and stress first. Some doctors use a variety of supplements to lower cortisol, such as natural herbs and ashwagandha. Once this is done, you can start testosterone replacement therapy. If your cortisol levels are too high, this will interfere with your treatment, as both cortisol and testosterone compete with each other. As I told you, hormones must work together, like a symphony. No amount of testosterone will help you if you do not address your stress. If you drink too much alcohol, testosterone can break down into estrogen too, the female sex hormone, and you can develop enlarged men's breasts. Lifestyle choices make an enormous difference.

The testosterone treatments available today—such as sublingual lozenges, injectables, patches, creams, nasal sprays, and gels—can be quite effective and easy to use with minimal side effects. The benefits they offer include:

• Improved energy and overall well-being

- Increased strength and stamina
- Enhanced mood and self-esteem
- Improved concentration and memory
- Enhanced libido and sexual function

Foods and Supplements That Help Testosterone

Before you get a script from your doctor for testosterone replacement therapy, do your part. Testosterone-boosting foods include eggs, liver, butter, fish, poultry, animal products, and cholesterol-rich foods. Go organic if you can afford it. Also eat more seafood. Oysters are considered an aphrodisiac as they are rich in zinc, which supports testosterone. But zinc is present in all seafood; it does not have to be just oysters. To curtail the breakdown of testosterone to estrogen and give your treatment a boost, take 100 mg of zinc, 750 mg of bioflavonoid chrysin, and 7.5 mg of pipeline daily.

The Benefits of Healthy Levels of Testosterone

At the right levels, testosterone helps prevent heart and Alzheimer's diseases. Testosterone helps keep muscle and bone mass and strength as we age. It is also good for normal hair growth and libido.

Preserving Testosterone Levels as You Age

To keep your hormones functioning for as long as possible without treatment, remember how much your overall lifestyle choices affect your physical well-being. Keep this in mind:

- **Exercise.** Keep your weight at the right level. Carrying excess fat around is bad for your hormones, muscles, bones, and about everything else.
- **Stop smoking.** Smoking is not only bad for your testosterone, but it can also lead to premature aging, emphysema, and lung cancer. Smoking damages your DNA and your testicles' cells.

- **Limit alcohol.** A lot of daily drinking raises your insulin levels, shuts down your sex hormones, and makes you age faster. If you need help quitting, contact Alcoholics Anonymous or ask your doctor for medications that can help you quit.
- **Avoid drugs.** Recreational drugs mess up your sex hormones. Get help if you need to.
- **Get sunshine in the early morning or late afternoon.** Sun for twenty minutes daily as it supports vitamin D production. Vitamin D supports your sex hormones. Avoid the midday sun as it will quickly make you look years older.
- **Use red light therapy often.** Place a red light twelve inches away from your testicles. It can raise testosterone levels severalfold. You'll learn more about red light therapy in Chapter 20.

When Too Much of a Good Thing (Testosterone) Is Bad

Boosting testosterone naturally is good. Replacing testosterone if it is too low is also good, as low levels are linked to increased mortality. But elevated levels of testosterone beyond normal range are also bad. Exogenous testosterone, in excess, does not lead to an increase in lifespan or longevity. In fact, excess supplementation can shorten someone's life. You can have a heart attack as your body makes more red blood cells, which can lead to a clot. Think of athletes who abuse testosterone with no medical supervision. Hormones must be in the perfect range. It is certainly good to use some testosterone supplementation in moderation to get your youth and vitality back, but never do it on your own. If you have low testosterone, consult with an experienced doctor in testosterone replacement therapy.

Human Growth Hormone (HGH) and the Myth of Longevity

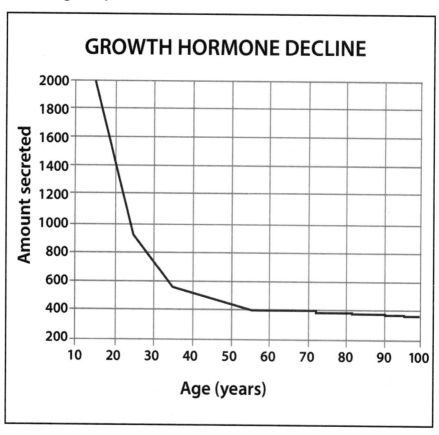

Now, we come to the biggest myth in the anti-aging arena, human growth hormone (HGH). Many doctors have been giving patients human growth hormone to fight aging for decades. Anti-aging clinics and anti-aging doctors that prescribe HGH are everywhere and popping up all over the country.

Doctors call HGH the fountain of youth. HGH helps to regulate body composition, body fluids, muscle and bone growth, sugar and fat metabolism, and possibly heart function. But natural human growth hormone production decreases steadily between ages twenty-five to thirty. That is when our bodies begin to show signs of aging—sagging skin, premature wrinkles, sluggish metabolism—and we cannot perform at our best level. Natural HGH is essential to our overall health, as well as our ability to lose weight and build muscle. It is still always best to stimulate your own natural production of HGH, and not to take it exogenously.

The Dangers of Exogenous HGH Administration

Many people inject HGH for longevity and to stay young longer. HGH is produced naturally by the pituitary gland and is particularly important for growth in children and adolescents. Without HGH, we would all be dwarfs. With too much, we would all be giants.

But if you inject synthetic HGH to fight aging, you are accelerating your aging process, and you could die prematurely!

Competitive athletes use of synthetic HGH leads to more stamina, stronger muscles, and weight loss. Their injuries heal faster. It is no wonder that the average person thinks it is a good idea to try this shortcut to strengthen muscles and have a fantastic-looking body. It turns out that, in fact, it is a terrible idea. HGH supplementation is a short-term fix for energy that leads to long-term problems.

When synthetic HGH is injected into the body, it can be overused, leading to an overdose. Side effects include premature aging, sore joints, carpal tunnel syndrome, insulin resistance, high blood pressure, edema, diabetes, heart disease, cancer, and early death. Exogenous HGH turns on the mTOR pathway. Remember, this is the elevator you do not want to overuse when you get older. HGH can also burn your telomeres. Hence, exogenous HGH negatively impacts the hallmarks of aging and can shorten your life.

I know I am going against those clinics and centers that are promising youth, but yes, injecting HGH can prematurely kill you. You need to slow down the mTOR pathway to live long. You also need to have long telomeres, not short ones.

HGH must be boosted naturally, by lifestyle. But do not take HGH exogenously unless you have a deficiency like a traumatic brain injury.

Addressing HGH Decline Naturally

HGH levels are disturbed by frequent meals, so the eat-every-three-hours approach is misguided. Instead reread the information on the intermittent fasting choices in Chapter 14. Fasting encourages HGH production and secretion. Intense physical exercise or anaerobic exercise increase HGH too.

The easiest way to increase your HGH naturally is to get a good night's sleep. As you drift into dreamland, 75 percent of your current HGH is secreted and absorbed by cells and organs. You'll find the suggestions about sleep I discussed earlier. And, of course, eat smart: poultry, eggs, fish, fruits, and vegetables. Do not eat anything two to three hours before bedtime.

When I was a guest on *The Dr. Oz Show* a few years ago, many guests on the show who were using HGH were praising how young they feel and how they look on this miraculous hormone. I said that I was against it unless there was a deficiency. I am still against the exogenous use of HGH unless there is a clear medical cause. I was right long before the hallmarks of aging were discovered.

If you are using HGH for longevity, get off it right now. Instead, maintain and increase your HGH level naturally. Bottom line? Do not fall for an easy way to stay young.

A Patient's Story

When Steve came to see me as a new patient in 2016, he was forty-eight years old, 5 feet 11 inches, and weighed 240 pounds. He complained of fatigue, unexplained weight gain, decreased libido, erection issues, and a depressed mood. His blood workups from previous doctors were all normal except for low testosterone levels that no one treated. In fact, he was told his testosterone was normal by three different doctors, since it fell right at 300 ng/dl.

His doctors told him it was part of getting older, and he was given a script for Viagra and an antidepressant. But Steve's symptoms were all consistent with low testosterone. Steve followed a low-fat diet and was missing many vitamins.

With the right diet, supplements, and testosterone replacement therapy, Steve lost seventy pounds in seventeen months. He now has the energy, sex drive, and erections of a man in his twenties.

Like Steve, you can get your youth and vitality back with natural hormone replacement. We no longer must take the same path as our parents and grandparents. We can age in a different way. It is time to bring vitality back into your life regardless of your age.

Remember . . .

- Take good care of your hormones by following a balanced natural diet and good lifestyle.

- *Bioidentical hormones* should be the go-to choice. Talk to your doctor about prescribing them if you need them. Natural hormones are now found at your local pharmacy and are covered by insurance.

- *Compounded bioidentical* hormones are made especially for you according to your specific needs.

- *Women's hormones* decrease and disappear after menopause. Estradiol is available in gel and vaginal cream. Progesterone should be taken or cream should be applied for only two weeks a month. If prescribed every day, it can lead to some weight gain. If your sex drive is lacking, you may need a small dose of testosterone.

- Testosterone replacement therapy is available in sublingual lozenges, nasal sprays, injectables, patches, creams, and gels. Increase your testosterone naturally. Take 100 mg of zinc, 750 mg flavonoid chrysin, and 7.5 mg piperine daily. Never use testosterone without the advice of your doctor.

- *Lab tests* are not always reflective of your age. When your doctor gives you the results of your tests, ask him or her about the lab's reference ranges for your age. He or she might just stick to the "average" for your age, but the goal is to balance your hormones like a young person.

- *HGH* can be increased naturally by adjusting your eating habits. Try intermittent fasting and challenging exercise like anaerobic or even high-intensity interval training (HIIT).

- *HGH* is secreted at night, so sleep time of at least eight hours is essential for longevity.

CHAPTER 19

Breakthrough Medications for Longevity

You are never too old to become younger!
—Mae West

We live in the best times. Targeting the ten hallmarks of aging enables us to live healthier, longer lives. Imagine living in the 1500s. This was before the discovery of the microscope, which let us examine the cells closely. Or imagine living before Louis Pasteur proposed the germ theory. Think of all the women who died in childbirth in their twenties and thirties from septic techniques. Think of all the millions and millions of people who died from tuberculosis in the last few centuries including the ones who left cultural treasures: Jane Austen, Frederic Chopin, Molière, and Amedeo Modigliani.

The shift to modern medicine 2.0 in the late twentieth century was a long path that took millennia. The twentieth century was the century of invention of antibiotics and vaccines. Advances in medicine are happening at lightning speed. It took scientists two years only to come up with a Covid-19 vaccine once the pandemic happened. Medicine 3.0 will arrive when doctors start targeting the ten hallmarks of aging and treating aging as a disease because the secret of our longevity is buried in our DNA.

One of the problems in allopathic medical care is that we target old-age diseases on a separate basis. We have separate organizations like the American Heart Association, the American Cancer Society, and the Alzheimer's Association. All the efforts of these organizations are toward research and prevention of the disease they cover. But if we target the cells, via common drivers, we can target all diseases of aging all at once.

I think that the secret that all centenarians have in common comes down to one thing: resilience. They were able to resist heart disease, type 2 diabetes, cancer, and neurodegenerative diseases even when they have smoked for decades or did not eat healthy. In the end, 70 percent of how you age is up to you.

The Ageless Revolution: A Different Way to Age

Surprisingly, when I decided to write *The Ageless Revolution*, one of my patients said to me, "You are the problem, doctor, you are making people live forever! It is a burden on society!" I was disappointed to hear such a statement, especially since I had suggested some supplements that would help him with his cholesterol. But I can't blame him. The prevailing view that people who live longer are a burden on society is not true if that population is healthy. Older people can be very productive and work until the very end. We must disrupt the existing medical paradigm and the way we think.

The practice of medicine is now old-fashioned, stuck in the twentieth century. We need a model that challenges the status quo. We need molecular ways to target the DNA and new ways to manipulate aging. I know that my views would be considered unconventional by most people and even doctors. My answer is to become educated and do your research. Doing nothing about the hallmarks of aging now that we have the defenses against them is the definition of insanity.

I also know many of the anti-aging books that preceded me have catered to the people who have the means. I am starting a revolution to make this program accessible to everyone regardless of financial status. Simple lifestyle changes, a good diet, some supplements, and a few meds that are affordable, and you are on your way to becoming ageless. I want everyone to have a chance to live their best life now.

The Fountain of Youth in a Pill?

Wouldn't it be amazing if there were a pill or an injection that could turn back the clock? Fortunately, some medications are at this point or coming close.

But these medications may not always be covered by your insurance. Remember, *aging* is not a disease to the insurance companies. Doctors and insurance companies see *aging* as natural, a part of life.

If you pay out of pocket for those medications, of course, you will have to evaluate your priorities. What is important to you? Is it the newest cell phone with a better camera or a two-year supply of a medication that can extend your life? Is it one fancy meal at a three-star Michelin restaurant or a year's supply of a drug that can make you live longer? You get the point as I can hear some who will say, "This is expensive, Doc." Personally, I am happy to pay $2,000 a year on supplements and medications that can extend my life for years. Of course if I lived in Sardinia and did my 10,000 steps a day and ate foraged food, I would not have to spend a dime. But I don't. My diet is not perfect even when I try to do my very best. I live in New York, where everyone seems stressed and running. This is the perfect recipe to kill everyone, even the immortals. Luckily, these advances are quite cheap and within the budget of most people. But here is the problem: you will need a prescription from a doctor who practices functional medicine and is experienced working with these breakthrough medications. You may feel a little overwhelmed by the number of medications discussed, but you don't need all of them; I just want you to be informed.

Metformin: The Best Anti-Aging Drug Available

Optimizing cell pathways fights aging, and metformin, from the French lilac flower, can help. Back in 1918, a scientist discovered that one of metformin's ingredients, guanidine, helps lower blood sugar, but this discovery fell out of favor after insulin was discovered. Metformin also helps with pre-diabetes, polycystic ovary syndrome, and weight gain. So, what does a diabetes drug have to do with anti-aging?

Metformin is the best anti-aging drug we have for now. It works on the AMPK pathway, one of the nutrient pathways that I compared to the elevator in the hotel, which slows down as we age. Remember, deregulated nutrient sensing is one of the ten hallmarks of aging. Metformin fixes this pathway. It's like a mechanic that fixes that elevator.

Metformin reduces the incidence of aging-related diseases such as neurodegenerative disease, heart disease, stroke, and cancer. Despite its widespread use, all the mechanisms by which metformin works on aging remain unknown. Further, not all individuals prescribed metformin derive the same benefits, and some develop side effects. Those side effects can include abdominal pain, bloating, diarrhea, nausea, and vomiting. Lactic acidosis is rare, but patients with severe renal and liver dysfunction are more at risk. Monitoring B12 blood levels is essential since they can become depleted.

Metformin may cancel out some exercise benefits. A small study showed a loss of less than 5 percent of muscle mass produced due to metformin, but the results are not conclusive. This may have to do with the fact that people who took metformin do less repetitive movements during their workout.

Dihydroberberine, a supplement I discussed earlier that you can buy over the counter, may give you the same benefits as metformin, and it does not cancel exercise. But no human longevity studies on dihydroberberine are available.

If you want to take metformin, you'll need to find a doctor (often one who practices functional medicine) who understands aging and is willing to give you a prescription when you do not have diabetes. Most doctors are reluctant to give metformin to nondiabetic patients as an anti-aging drug. Unfortunately, most doctors will tell you, "Your sugar is normal; you do not need it." The good news is that there are a few doctors who know the benefits of metformin and will prescribe it for anti-aging purposes.

Metformin is safe and inexpensive. A script for sixty tablets is like ten to thirty dollars. You can take metformin starting from age forty, especially if you are prediabetic. Start slow, at 500 mg orally a day. If you cannot tolerate it, or have abdominal pain, ask your doctor to switch you to the extended-release type. If you are concerned about muscle buildup, skip metformin on the days you do an anaerobic activity. Eventually, you can increase the dose from 500 mg to 1–2 grams a day. Do not take metformin if you have any kidney issues. I take both my supplements and my metformin. I wouldn't be caught dead without them.

Acarbose

You only need metformin or acarbose, not both. But acarbose is also worth discussing. The good news, it is also very inexpensive. It is less than seventeen dollars for thirty tablets. The National Institute on Aging Interventions Testing Program (ITP) was designed to be the most exhaustive testing framework and system that evaluates whether longevity molecules extend longevity in mice and to understand the underlying mechanisms that lead to this benefit. One of the drugs studied for longevity is another diabetes drug called acarbose. Acarbose works by slowing the action of certain chemicals so less sugar is absorbed in the bloodstream. The ITP showed that acarbose led to an increase in lifespan in the animal model they were studying, especially when acarbose was combined with another drug called rapamycin that I will discuss later on.

Unfortunately, we have no human studies on acarbose, but it looks like acarbose impacts longevity in animals through several mechanisms. It affects the gut flora, it lowers inflammation, lengthens telomeres, and supports mitochondria. The dose for longevity in humans is unknown. Some biohackers take 25 mg of acarbose two to three times a day.

Low-Dose Naltrexone (LDN)

As you've learned, it's important to get rid of the zombie cells that impair our bodies as we age because they secrete toxins. This can be done with intermittent fasting, supplements like fisetin, or by taking low-dose naltrexone. Some biohackers take this drug.

Although used for inflammatory diseases for forty years, using low-dose naltrexone (LDN) to promote longevity and health is comparatively new. In the late 1980s, Dr. Bernard Bihari noted that AIDS patients had endorphin levels that were much lower than normal and connected this to their lower immunity. Endorphins are polypeptides produced by the pituitary gland and central nervous system that regulate the production of neurotransmitters like dopamine and serotonin. As Dr. Bihari researched medications that would raise endorphin levels, he came upon naltrexone. When he delved deeper, he found it could help AIDS patients fight off opportunistic infections and live longer.

Since then, naltrexone has been used to treat fibromyalgia, Crohn's disease, multiple sclerosis, rheumatoid arthritis, chronic fatigue, obesity, and chronic pain. Naltrexone's endorphin boost can also treat mood disorders like anxiety, depression, and post-traumatic stress disorder (PTSD).

What do many of these illnesses have in common? They are driven by inflammation. Yes, even some forms of depression have been linked to mild inflammation. Inflammation and oxidative stress are common causes of early aging. This type of inflammation is called *inflammaging*. Low-dose naltrexone can get rid of senescent cells, the zombie cells, one of the ten hallmarks of aging. Like fisetin and quercetin, low-dose naltrexone helps to get rid of those senescent cells.

LDN boosts the body's natural production of endorphins, which play a role in stimulating other elements to decrease oxidative stress. Endorphins help reduce pain and inflammation and promote autophagy and cellular cleanup. Side effects are mild on such a low dose. Vivid dreams, sleep disturbance, mild increase in anxiety, headaches, and nausea subside within a few days if they pop up at all. Eating a vegetable-abundant diet helps LDN work at its best. To get low-dose naltrexone, you will need to get a prescription from a doctor who understands aging. The dose is 4.5 mg daily of LDN, preferably taken at bedtime. The good news is that LDN is very inexpensive. It is about forty dollars for thirty tablets.

Dasatinib

There are multiple ways to get rid of the zombie cells; you only need one choice. I gave you plenty of choices. Dasatinib is a cancer drug sold under the brand name Sprycel. It is another drug that can get rid of senescent cells. Of course, intermittent fasting is the safest and cheapest way. But what does a cancer drug have to do with longevity? Animal studies, but no peer-reviewed studies, show that dasatinib eliminates senescent cells when taken with quercetin. Doses up to 100 mg a day appear to be safe. Doctors who prescribe this drug usually give it a dose of less than 500 mg a day because it can come with some serious side effects, including low blood-cell counts, anemia, rash, bleeding, pulmonary edema, and heart failure. I prefer safer drugs and options to eliminate senescent cells.

GLP-1 Peptides for Weight Loss

There has been a revolution in weight-loss drugs in the last few years: new weight-loss drugs that are a game changer in the obesity epidemic. From Oprah to Sharon Osbourne, everyone seems to be taking one of those drugs. They do magic when nothing else works. So if you are overweight, your first goal on *The Ageless Revolution* should be to lose those excess pounds. Yes, you can do it with the right diet and exercise, but some medications can give a boost to lose all the weight you want if you have a hard time. These drugs should be a last resort. In addition, these drugs are super expensive even when compounded.

When you eat, insulin is secreted, and this tells your brain that you're hungry and to store nutrients as fat. Glucagon-like peptides (GLP) are a collection of amino acids that tell your brain you are full.

These drugs have broad pharmacological potentials, decrease in gastric emptying, and inhibit food intake. For this reason, these peptides are used for both the treatment of diabetes and for weight loss.

GLP-1 medications are used for the treatment of obesity, a disease associated with many complications. Weight loss of 5 to 15 percent can improve many obesity-related complications.

The prevalence of obesity in the United States and the Western world has been increasing over the past few decades, and despite the availability of approved anti-obesity medications (AOMs), people with obesity may not be accessing or receiving treatment at levels consistent with the disease prevalence.

Because of their effectiveness in reducing body weight, a daily subcutaneous injection of liraglutide 3.0 mg (Saxenda) has been approved by the FDA in 2014. But it wasn't a very good drug. More effective weight loss came from another peptide called semaglutide (Ozempic). It is administered once weekly by subcutaneous administration. Later on, tirzepatide came on the market.

People have been flocking to doctors' offices for peptides such as semaglutide (Wegovy), oral semaglutide (Rybelsus), and tirzepatide (Mounjaro) or (Zepbound).

Tirzepatide appears to be the most effective GLP drug for weight loss on the market now. Retatrudie is another GLP drug under investigation and is expected to be approved in two years. It is called Triple G as it works on three hormones that affect satiety. It is so strong that people lost one third of their body weight when they took it.

The doses of those drugs vary and are adjusted to the patient's needs. These peptides are highly effective in allowing people to lose tons of weight, which can add years to their life. Those GLP-1 peptides also have cardio and neuroprotective effects because they decrease inflammation. Again, they should be a last resort. The right diet and exercise should always be the first steps.

A prescription from your doctor is needed, along with clear instructions on how to use these peptides. The cost may be covered by your insurance plan depending on your weight and body mass index if it's over twenty-six.

Start slow at the lowest dose possible to avoid side effects that can include bloating, nausea, and vomiting. There is also an increased risk for clots. You lose fat, but muscle mass as well anytime you lose weight, so make sure to include anaerobic activity if you take one of those drugs. There are reports of face wasting, or Ozempic face, related to fast weight loss as seen on TikTok. But it's not related to those peptides.

Instead, lose weight slowly, like one pound a week, to allow your skin not to be saggy. These drugs may be contraindicated if you have a history of thyroid cancer, but this is based on animal studies so far, not human cases.

As you have seen, there are many drugs that can affect longevity. It all depends on your medical needs. I take metformin. Some people take acarbose. Some people need to lose weight, so they take GLP-1 peptides. The right doctor can guide you in your ageless journey.

Remember . . .

- Discuss the anti-aging medications that you feel are appropriate with your primary doctor.

- *Metformin*, a diabetes medicine, also reduces age-related neurodegenerative diseases like heart disease, stroke, and cancer even in nondiabetics.

- *Acarbose*, a diabetes drug, may also help with longevity.

- *Low-dose naltrexone* fights fibromyalgia, Crohn's disease, multiple sclerosis, rheumatoid arthritis, alcohol addiction, chronic fatigue, obesity, and chronic pain. It boosts endorphins and decreases oxidative stress. It does the same job as fisetin and quercetin, which can be purchased over the counter.

- *Dasatinib* is a cancer drug that kills senescent cells. Use safer supplements.

- GLP-1 peptides are used for weight loss. They can also decrease cardiovascular risk, stroke, and cardiovascular death. They may be covered by your insurance if you are overweight. They should be your last resort.

- Ozempic, aka Wegovy (Semaglutide), is a weight-loss peptide given once a week.

- Mounjaro, aka Zepbound (Tirzepatide), appears to be the most effective GLP drug for weight loss on the market now.

CHAPTER 20

Looking Ageless at Any Age

Beauty is about enhancing what you have.
—Janelle Mona

Call me vain, call me superficial, but I also want to look good as I get older. There have been many advances in dermatology—it is possible to have more collagen and less wrinkles at an older age. Have you ever wondered why so many Hollywood stars look young and have glowing skin even at an older age? Those movie stars claim they just eat right and sleep well. They do that, but they have a lot of help from personal trainers, chefs, and nutritionists. They also have access to the best plastic surgeons, and cosmetic dermatologists money can buy and can afford expensive and unconventional treatments for their skin. In fact, they are already doing many of the things I discuss in *The Ageless Revolution*. So I will discuss in this chapter the advances happening in skin care but on a budget. Again, I wrote *The Ageless Revolution* for everyone.

The good news is you can improve your skin's appearance and age on the cellular level. There are two aspects for aging skin: laxity and texture. There is nothing to do about laxity except for surgeries. Lasers may help a little. Those options are usually reserved for the ones with the means, those who can afford them. But you can control your skin texture with good and cheap skin care, and without breaking the bank.

Addressing Skin Laxity with Facelifts

Starting in our twenties, we begin to lose collagen. How sad is that! With time, we eventually look old. For skin laxity, I am afraid the only thing that can truly help is—facelifts. That's an expensive option that many of us can't afford. It is also beyond the scope of this book that deals with cellular health. Of course, a facelift is camouflage. It does not change your cells. If you have the means, you will have to find the right surgeon. The first facelift was performed in 1901 by a German surgeon. It removed the excess skin. The results were an unnatural pulled look, non-lasting as the problem is in the fascia, which is the layer under the skin. This traditional old-approach facelift is still the one performed by most plastic surgeons.

In the 1950–1970s, newer techniques that addressed the fascia were introduced. This led to the introduction of deep plane facelifts in the 1980s, which pulled the fascia under the skin. This facelift addresses the midface. Although deep plane facelifts have been around for decades, very few doctors know how to do them. The surgeon needs to know the facial anatomy and have the experience. They are quite expensive.

Nothing happened for decades until a plastic surgeon in San Diego named Dr. Amir Karam came up with a revolutionary approach a few years ago. It is called vertical restore. Dr. Karam's technique addresses the whole face and neck. It lifts the skin and fascia with a deep plane approach but upward since with age our skin goes down. This facelift technique addresses the whole face and gives the most dramatic and natural results you can imagine. Many doctors followed in his footsteps as they started to lift the face up. It truly revolutionized facelifts with the most natural results in this century. Of course, facelifts are options for the ones with the means, so let's move on to skin texture.

Home Procedures for Skin Texture

Light Therapy (Blue, White, and Green)

Light therapy is among the earliest recorded healing modalities. Solar therapy was used by the ancient Egyptians, and light therapy was practiced by the ancient Chinese, Greeks, and East Indians. Research shows how different wavelengths affect the body at the cellular level. Light therapy is noninvasive, nonthermal, and without side effects. Instead of spending money to see a dermatologist for a laser treatment, try this instead.

Lamps that you can buy online come in red, blue, white, and green—each with special and similar results. All are effective anti-aging treatments because they repair skin damage.

All these colors emit different wavelengths on the electromagnetic spectrum. For example, blue has a shorter wavelength and higher frequency than red light. Blue light therapy improves skin texture, reduces enlarged oil glands, and is commonly used for acne. Do not confuse the blue light in those devices with the dangerous blue light from your phone or tablet.

White light therapy is more effective in treating symptoms of depression than red light. It also tightens the skin, heals acne scars, reduces inflammation, and clears sun damage. Green light is, like the others, an anti-aging treatment. It improves skin pigmentation due to overexposure to the sun's UV rays, improves sleep, and treats seasonal affective disorder.

Depending on your skin needs, you can also buy a light mask online, which comes in all colors including red. Use it two or three times a week for twenty minutes for each session. It might cost $100–$200, but it is certainly cheaper than expensive laser treatments at your cosmetic dermatologist that could run you a few thousands dollars. It has less dramatic results, but it is something you can continue doing on your own on this journey to becoming ageless.

Red Light Therapy (RLT) and Infrared Light

Buying a red-light panel is the best investment you can make after eating right, intermittent fasting, and exercising. Use red light therapy for more youthful skin or a fuller head of hair. Red light therapy (RLT) stimulates the regeneration of the skin because the light emitted by RLT penetrates five millimeters below the skin's surface.

Red light therapy is quite different from the red light emitted by tanning beds that were popular in the 1980s. Those dangerous tanning beds emitted UV rays, which can lead to skin cancer.

Red light beds may help reduce wrinkles and stretch marks. In the medical field, they are used to treat psoriasis, eczema, slow-healing wounds like foot ulcers, and side effects of chemotherapy.

It's possible that this light may strengthen damaged mitochondria chromophores when photons are released in skin cells. This increases blood flow and oxygen absorption.

Adenosine triphosphate (ATP) nitric acid release spurs biological reactions that energize cells to function more efficiently, rejuvenate themselves, and repair damage.

Red light therapy is like a wake-up call for your cells, and it cleans up the debris. You can buy red light panels for the face and larger panels for the entire body. They even come in helmets for people who want to grow their hair or in face masks for those who want glowing skin.

Make sure to use a brand that has fire-bright red light and infrared at 850 nm waves. If you cannot afford red light therapy, I suggest using an infrared sauna blanket.

But to get the look of the movie stars without spending a fortune, there is another solution. Buy a forty-watt LED red light bulb. Use it over your skin or scalp and use some eye protectors. Now you have your own red light home unit for forty dollars or less!

Professional Microneedling

For those with some means, and for a fraction of the cost of facelifts, some lasers and some microneedling can help a little with skin laxity. They can also help with texture and collagen buildup. Who wouldn't love that! The bad news, this procedure can run you a few hundred bucks a session. It is done at your dermatologist or plastic surgeon's office. The good thing is it is not camouflage. You are building your collagen bank. For this procedure, a numbing cream is applied to the face. After thirty to forty minutes, small needles penetrate the skin to injure it, new cells are formed a few months after. When you injure your skin, new collagen is formed. Three forms of microneedling exist. Microneedling can be done with a simple microneedling pen (mechanical injury) or with microneedling and radiofrequency (mechanical and heat injury) Or it can be done with a roller at home. I advocate against home microneedling as you can get infections. The needles do not go deep enough. Check out those procedures at a medical professional near you if you can afford them. When your skin is injured, the cells release growth factors to heal the injuries. This method has shown positive results. You will see fewer wrinkles and better-looking skin long term.

Have you ever heard of the "vampire" facial? Kim Kardashian brought this facial into the spotlight in 2013 when she shared scary post-procedure photos of herself on social media with blood splashed all over her face at her doctor's office. For this facial, blood is drawn from your own veins, then spun in a centrifuge to isolate the natural growth factors. A topical anesthesia is applied on the face, left for thirty minutes, cleaned, and then your face is microneedled.

Blood will be oozing out of the skin from all the deep pores produced. The platelet-rich plasma, or PRP, with important growth factors is rubbed or injected back into areas of your face to restore the growth of new cells. The platelet-rich plasma is called a gold elixir because it is so rich in growth factors. You will probably need several sessions of microneedling with PRP to see positive skin results. Another way to magnify the results of microneedling is to use exosomes.

Exosomes can be injected or rubbed into your face after microneedling to help build new collagen and result in glowing skin.

Remember stem cells, or Plastic Man? The cells can be turned into any kind of cells you need. Stem cells deliver their message via exosomes, which are extracellular vehicles that carry RNA, micro-RNA, and proteins including growth factors.

Think of exosomes like the FedEx delivery or mail carrier who delivers the mail or messages. Although exosomes are considered noncellular material, at reputable labs, tissue donors are screened for HIV and both hepatitis B and C before exosomes are harvested, primarily for testing new medical treatments. The results of this procedure have proven very positive. When they are injected into the skin for rejuvenation, it is theorized that the exosomes target the existing stem cells there. Again, they can also be rubbed on the skin after microneedling or injected to improve complexion and collagen repair.

Exosome treatment combined with microneedling and PRP are much more effective than PRP alone for skin rejuvenation and hair growth. Yes, exosome treatments are expensive because it takes a lot of work to harvest the exosomes. In general, billions or trillions of exosomes need to be injected into the skin by a professional experienced in microneedling.

Many advances from red light to microneedling can help turn back time. For a fraction of the cost of facelifts, we can have glowing skin as we age.

Sculpting Your Body

Emsculpt Neo

Many people can't exercise due to neck or back injuries, or a debilitating illness, but you need to preserve your muscles as you get old. What can you do if you can't work out? Discover Emsculpt Neo. It is a machine that tricks your body into working without stepping food in a gym. Emsculpt Neo is an aesthetic device to build muscles in a short thirty-minute session. It works by high intensity electromagnetic therapy and can firm muscles through automatic contractures. The machine also has a radiofrequency unit built in, so it melts fat too. It is a double benefit to get stronger and be leaner. You can find those machines at your doctor's office and high-end spas, but the sessions are quite expensive and can run you a few thousand dollars. Four sessions are usually needed to see results. But if you have an injury and cannot exercise, this may be an option. Again, this is a costly procedure but can be an option for those who can afford it and want to build muscles without working out. I will offer an alternative to the expensive Emsculpt Neo; it is called Power Plat. It will be discussed in the next chapter.

I have tried to give answers for most people reading this book. I use my red light frequently, and I occasionally get a laser or microneedling done on my face once or twice a year. Don't overdo it. Give your face the time to heal after such injuries to build collagen. These measures with good skin care using vitamin C, retinoic acid, and niacinamide have given me great results. They are cheap. No need for expensive luxury creams from big brands with alcohol, parabens, and chemicals. Skin care as we get older should be simple. Take care of your body on the inside and the outside with all the affordable measures discussed in this book.

Remember . . .

- There are several new cellular skin anti-aging possibilities that can be done at home, such as red light.

- For skin use *light therapy* in red, white, and blue. Check websites for units that offer red light with 850 nm wavelengths. You can buy a cap or helmet that has light therapy to help reverse hair loss.

- For young-looking skin try *exosome treatments* after microneedling, done in wellness centers and by knowledgeable doctors.

- For your entire body, *infrared light beds* are becoming popular in spas, and some specialized facilities are in malls and shopping centers. Do not confuse them with the old UV tanning beds!

- Try professional microneedling if you can afford it to build collagen.

CHAPTER 21

A Glimpse into the Future

Age is no barrier.
It's a limitation you put on your mind.
—Jackie Joyner-Kersee

I hope my book has given you hope that you can age in a new healthy way. Simple measures like the right diet and exercise must be your first steps in this journey. Supplements and medications must be your next stop. This chapter is indeed futuristic, but many of these advances and measures are already here. Medicine is advancing rapidly, and the field of anti-aging is moving at lightning speed. This chapter investigates how advanced and regenerative medicine can help turn back the clock in terms of chronic diseases in new ways that you may never have imagined. Some of these measures are hard to find, but I want to give answers and hope to everyone reading this book. There is always hope. In fact, with my Nostradamus hat on, I see many of those advances being readily available in the future.

Enhanced External Counterpulsation (EECP)

Have a circulation issue? Discover EECP. As we get older, many of our issues, conditions such as congestive heart failure, stroke, hypertension, and renal disease are circulatory in nature. Enhanced External Counterpulsation, or EECP, enhances blood circulation and increases collateral flow in the same way that exercise does.

During this drug-free, advanced procedure, the patient lies on the table and is wrapped with blood pressure cuffs. A generator is used to inflate and deflate the cuffs, and an EKG is also used to track the heart rate. Over a period of several sessions and weeks, new blood vessels are formed. EECP helps with kidney flow, blood pressure, and erectile dysfunction. EECP also improves blood flow to the heart as it squeezes the blood from the leg to the heart. This procedure is FDA approved and may be covered by most insurance. There are no contraindications. If you have a circulatory issue with EECP, try to find doctors who offer this procedure in your area.

Exercise with Oxygen Therapy (EWOT)

Want more energy? Have sleep issues? Need faster results from your workouts? If you don't want to use medications, discover EWOT. There are many fancy gyms that already offer this service. The goal of exercise with oxygen therapy is to breathe higher concentrations of pure oxygen during workouts.

To do this you use oxygen concentrators to increase purity such as a mask or nasal cannula. This allows you to breathe in high purity oxygen from the machine while, say, using the treadmill. While the air we breathe contains oxygen, this extra oxygen can improve energy, mood, and concentration. This type of exercise can lead to reduced stress, fewer headaches, enhanced athletic performance, and improved sleep. Professional athletes are already using oxygen during exercise to improve their performance. They do it for no more than fifteen minutes while on a treadmill or a stationary bike. When done correctly and for no more than fifteen minutes at a time, there are no risks or side effects from exercising with oxygen therapy. Breathing higher levels of oxygen is considered safe and there is no risk of oxygen toxicity. However, an oxygen tank can run you three thousand dollars. So this anti-aging trick may not be possible for many of us. Be on the lookout for this at your local gym as this procedure becomes more mainstream.

Power Plate

Have you lost muscle mass as you got older and can't seem to gain muscle quickly? Have chronic pain? If you can't afford Emsculpt Neo, no worries, discover Power Plate. It won't cost you a thing, just find a gym that has it. Power Plate is a machine that vibrates while you work out. You stand on a machine that vibrates while you take different positions. It is already at my local gym; I use it, and I love it.

Scientists have found that a Power Plate workout recruits 95 percent of your muscle fibers while a regular workout is shown to only recruit 55 percent. The 1,200 waves of energy every thirty seconds flow through your tendons, helping to remove all chronic pain over time. This machine also helps raise a newly discovered hormone called irisin, which is secreted by the muscles as it helps burn fat. It may also help with the conversion of white fat, which is bad, to brown fat, which is good and is present in younger people.

In addition, it helps raise growth hormone by a factor of four or five, which makes your entire physical system work better—the ultimate physical biohack! That exercise means that sitting, standing, or lying on a vibrating platform for ten minutes a day could be just as effective as huffing and puffing while lifting weights or going for a sweaty run. Try to join a gym that has these.

Hyperbaric Oxygen Chambers

One of my patients a few years ago had a diabetic foot ulcer, he was on the verge of gangrene, or death of the tissues. The ulcer wouldn't heal. A surgeon suggested a foot amputation, but I suggested a hyperbaric oxygen chamber. He did a few sessions, and the ulcer healed. No surgery or foot amputation was needed. It changed his life.

If you've had a traumatic brain injury, suffered severe burns or a transient ischemic attack, or have diabetic ulcers, look into hyperbaric oxygen chambers. They are used to help divers recover from decompression sickness, but scientists are discovering their many benefits include anti-aging. Hyperbaric oxygen chambers are an expensive and impractical option for most people for anti-aging. It is about sixty dollars a session. Michael Jackson used it after his scalp burn while filming a Pepsi commercial and other athletes and celebrities like Michael Phelps, LeBron James, Tiger Woods, Justin Bieber, Usher, Jennifer Aniston, Sylvester Stallone, and many more use them too.

Research on hyperbaric oxygen dates to the 1970s. Hyperbaric oxygen chambers involve breathing oxygen in a pressurized environment like being on a plane. Hyperbaric oxygen chambers can also improve age-related memory loss. A 2020 study in *Aging* magazine found that hyperbaric oxygen increased telomere length by 20 percent and decreased immunosenescence —the gradual deterioration of the immune system—in isolated red blood cells. Hyperbaric oxygen is beneficial for those with transient ischemic attacks, post strokes, Alzheimer's, and Parkinson's disease by increasing the blood flow and forming new blood vessels in the brain.

If you undergo treatment, the recommendation is for five (ninety-minute) sessions per week for twelve weeks.

If you are planning to have stem cells injected in your joints, it is a good idea to do hyperbaric oxygen for twenty sessions before the stem cells are extracted.

Stem Cells and Exosomes

Stem cells and exosomes are the buzzwords now in anti-aging. Doctors are using them in skin rejuvenation and joint issues. As you've learned, stem cells are non-differentiated cells, and they can become any cells you want them to be. Exhaustion of stem cells is one of the ten hallmarks of aging. By the time we are sixty or seventy, we run out of stem cells. Lifestyle choices including eating more dark chocolate, drinking black tea, and avoiding sugar can help your stem cells stay around longer. But when serious health issues arise, autologous, which means extracting stem cells from the blood, bone marrow, or fat, is an option. These are then reinjected where they are needed. Some people even bank their own stem cells when they are young as a form of insurance to use when they are old. Yes, there are banks for that. You deposit your stem cells when you are young. Stem cells communicate via exosomes, on a cell-to-cell level, and act as vehicles that deliver messages, like the UPS or the FedEx person who delivers packages.

Exosomes reprogram the receiving stem cells with their carried bioactive compounds to make them differentiate and work. As we age, stem cells become less effective, so exosomes can help. Exosomes improve signaling between cells, reduce inflammation, cause cells to regenerate, and change the body's immune response when it is no longer healthy. Exosomes tell cells to turn on or off certain functions, or to react in a certain way, for example, by telling stem cells to rush to an injury site and begin repairing tissue.

At present, in the United States, both stem cells and exosomes are not approved for any use except with some blood cancers. But many doctors are using them in rejuvenating skin treatment by microneedling or injecting them into the scalp for hair growth. They are also heavily used in orthopedic practices with positive results.

Can stem cells and exosomes be injected intravenously to give us youth and revitalize our cells? We will have to wait and see. It's so difficult to find those doctors who are willing to use these treatments for regeneration or anti-aging with all the FDA rules that ban unproven methods. As a result, people with serious medical conditions or for anti-aging have to travel abroad. Clinics in foreign countries do offer these regenerative treatments for serious illnesses, anti-aging, and—yes—rejuvenation.

In these clinics, stem cells and exosomes are injected into the spinal cord to reverse Lou Gehrig's disease. In certain cases, a patient with this deadly disease can live for a year or more with fewer symptoms after getting stem cell treatments. It is no cure, but it is progress. How about anti-aging! I believe that stem cells and exosomes can do magic for us and make us young again on the cellular level. However, human studies on stem cells and exosomes are still in their infancy.

But maybe one day instead of stopping at Starbucks to get an espresso shot, we will stop at a doctor's office to get a different intravenous shot of stem cells or exosomes: a shot that gives us youth.

Rapamycin

What if there is a drug that you can take to make you live to be 120 to 140 years old? Would you take that? You already know I love metformin, but rapamycin may be my second most favorite drug for anti-aging. Autophagy or recycling dead cell parts is essential for life. Imagine if you stopped taking the garbage out of your house, your house would soon become uninhabitable. By cleaning the damaged parts of the cells, autophagy allows the cells to run efficiently. This brings me to the most successful anti-aging drug ever discovered, rapamycin.

The discovery of this drug was purely accidental. Most people know about Easter Island because of the giant stone heads erected on the shoreline, called moai. The island was named by European explorers who landed on Easter Sunday in 1722, but the natives called the island Rapa Nui. Rapamycin was first identified in bacteria found on the island. Initially, it was used to develop a drug that prevented transplanted organs from being rejected. About thirty years later, researchers noticed that one of rapamycin's effects (admittedly on worms and yeast) was increased lifespan.

Researchers moved up the food chain to mice and found that the lifespans of the mice were increased to the equivalent of 140 years old in humans. Wow. Can we even beat the age, 122 years, of the French supercentenarian Jeanne Calment with rapamycin?

Although there is not a single supplement on the market that can truly claim to be the fountain of youth, rapamycin comes the closest to this claim. Technically, rapamycin is a controlled substance, a drug. But when used as a supplement, it can promote longevity. It is one of the most highly studied and researched drugs today because it improves the way that DNA is stored within our cells.

When DNA degenerates, we age; it is one of the ten hallmarks of aging. Rapamycin strengthens and encourages the growth of proteins that allow our DNA to remain intact and our cells to form chromosomes. Rapamycin can renew the energy of long-working, aging DNA cells.

That increase allows cell growth that not only prevents further aging but reverses it. Rapamycin also mimics the anti-aging benefits that are only gained from severe calorie restriction. It acts to mimic the effect of prolonged fasting.

Rapamycin may also be able to slow down the increase of age-related senescent cells. I talked earlier about how high-protein/low-carb diets and keto diets induce mTOR and increase the risk of early death. Rapamycin does the opposite. Rapamycin slows down the mTOR pathway that we need to use less as we get older.

Rapamycin binds directly to mTOR (complex 1) to encourage cellular autophagy. This means it gets rid of the zombie cells. With mTOR, rapamycin inhibits the growth signals that create senescent cells, reduces their inflammatory molecules (SASP), and shields healthy cells from turning into senescent ones.

As we age, we accumulate more senescent cells that are damaged or dying. Those zombie cells, neither fully alive nor completely dead, secrete toxins, a brew of inflammatory cytokines, chemokines, and proteases, resulting in a pro-inflammatory state. Rapamycin is a powerful inducer of autophagy, the body's evolutionary self-preservation system that removes dysfunctional cells and toxic proteins responsible for many age-related chronic diseases. It also recycles parts of them to repair and clean so that they keep working. Rapamycin silences the hypergrowth signals of senescent cells and curbs the number of toxins that are produced.

I've mentioned rapamycin in *The Ageless Revolution* for reference, as to date, we have no human studies on longevity. It is quite controversial. Those human studies can take decades. So is it safe? There are also serious side effects including elevated sugar levels resulting in pseudo diabetes and immuno-suppression if taken daily. But researchers also found that when taken weekly, it boosts the immune function.

More clinical trials are needed to find the right dosing of rapamycin so it can do its longevity job. Right now, there are some individuals who feel there is enough proof behind the relative safety of rapamycin and they take it intermittently, not daily. We will have to wait for further research to establish rapamycin's safety.

While dosage and efficacy of rapamycin are debated, it is still possible to get it prescribed by a knowledgeable doctor. But no one knows, yet, the right dose for longevity.

I personally take rapamycin at a minimal dose once a week, and I don't know if it will help me. I decided to be a guinea pig based on all the animal studies that were positive. It is risky, but I do know that aging can hurt me more than any side effects that this dose of rapamycin can ever give me. I monitor my sugar. Rapamycin is controversial, but doctors in the anti-aging arena are discovering that some supplements like hesperidin, gynostemma leaf extract, and intermittent fasting work on the same AMPK pathway. They are much safer. If you optimize this pathway with diet and metformin, the mTOR pathway is inhibited, and rapamycin may not even be needed.

Cells and Gene Therapy

Cells are the building blocks of living things. Genes are small sections of our DNA. Every person has around 2,000 genes and two copies of each of their genes—one from each parent. Variations in genes result in variations in people's appearance and potential health.

Genetic diseases happen when a critical section of the DNA is deleted, substituted, or duplicated. Can we insert part of the gene that the cell is missing or that is defective? Gene therapy has been used in cystic fibrosis, hemophilia, and sickle cell anemia. This process is only in the experimental stages, but it can be done by an adenovirus, which changes the segment of the DNA that is defective. This is very risky as adenovirus is very inflammatory, so these types of treatments are currently reserved for people with terminal illnesses or those who have no other choice.

However, this is an exciting advance because it changes the way we look at disease and may be able to treat genetic diseases in the future. Or even aging! What if we can alter our genes and make them become young with gene therapy again? No one knows. But let us hope this future happens in our lifetimes.

Cell therapy has been used by placing pancreatic cells to treat diabetes and corneal repairs. It is used to treat diseases by restoring sets of cells. They can be from the patient or from a donor. However, this cell therapy to replace a damaged part of our body is still a futuristic treatment in the anti-aging field.

Peptides

I take you now to Russia, to bring you the latest treatments in anti-aging—peptides, which are chains of amino acids or proteins bound together. Peptides are tiny but mighty molecules already running through your body. They deliver messages and nudge specific hormones and organs, reminding them to do their jobs. Some peptides have anti-aging effects.

Peptides are the new frontier in anti-aging. It is no wonder peptides are the new buzzword in the anti-aging medical community. Walk down any pharmacy aisle, and you will find a variety of skin creams that advertise that they contain peptides that will turn back the clock. But there is an injectable peptide that can make us live ten to twenty years. Peptide research played a military role during the Cold War (1945–1989). Professor Vladamir Khavinson was in the Soviet Union military, and his medical innovations with new peptide regulators served elite military units, cosmonauts, submarine crews exposed to nuclear reactors, and former residents of Chernobyl after the nuclear disaster there in 1986. Khavinson and other scientists continued longevity research to treat illnesses like Alzheimer's disease and other brain disorders, diabetes, and cancer. The research is mostly published in Russian, so few doctors in the United States know about peptides. It was Khavinson's work that brought epithalon, the brightest star peptide in anti-aging, into the spotlight. Epithalon is produced in the pineal gland. It can be given as an injection. It helps to protect DNA from damage by increasing the natural production of telomerase, the natural enzyme that helps cells reproduce telomeres. Remember, telomeres are often compared to the tips of shoelaces, a type of "cap" at the end of a DNA chromosome to keep it from fraying. DNA is a polymer of long chains of nucleotides. Telomerase is the enzyme that adds nucleotides to telomeres to make them longer and, therefore, stronger. Epithalon makes chromosomes longer. It also promotes deeper sleep, improves skin health and appearance, acts as an antioxidant, heals injuries and deteriorating muscle cells, and delays and prevents some age-related diseases like cancer, heart disease, and dementia. Epithalon is usually given by injection. The FDA banned compounding of epithalon, but some anti-aging doctors still have access to it from manufacturers. I hope it comes back on the market soon for all doctors. It is administered twice a year.

Another star peptide in the anti-aging world is GHK-copper or GHK-cu. It comes in face creams and injections. When injected subcutaneously, GHK-cu peptide can help you have glowing skin as you age. But GHK also stimulates the release of stem cells.

A peptide that helps stem cells, who wouldn't love that! GHK-cu is a tripeptide that occurs naturally in the copper complex found in human plasma, saliva, and urine. It is made of three amino acids—glycine-histidine-lysine—that are complexed with a copper molecule. GHK goes down with age, and when it does, there is a noticeable decrease in the regenerative ability of an organism. GHK-cu is also no longer available after a recent FDA ban. But some doctors have it from manufacturers. I hope it comes back soon.

My last peptide may be the most controversial peptide in anti-aging, and no one knows its long-term effects. Growth differentiation factor 11 (or GDF-11) is a powerful senolytic and antioxidant peptide that can repair stem cells. As we age, stem cells accumulate DNA damage, leading to stem cell senescence, the main characteristic of which is the decline in stem cell quantity and function. Exogenous GDF-11 can boost stem cells and the regenerative potential of the body, thereby reversing aging and improving the symptoms of age-related conditions. But as we age, levels of GDF-11 decline, which may be related to stem cell decline. Supplementing with GDF-11 keeps your stem cells young and regenerating. The discovery was also accidental. In 2013, a team of researchers found peptides in the blood of young mice. One of the peptide reversed age-related skeletal muscle and vascular and neurogenic function in the brain. It also reversed the symptoms of heart failure. It was related to GDF-11. In 2014, another paper labeled this peptide the fountain of youth.

Back in the 1950s, scientists experimented with connecting a young mouse to an old mouse, and the old mouse became young. We know now, this may be related to the abundance of GDF-11 in the younger mouse's blood. Avid biohackers took notice of this crazy old experiment, and some started getting blood transfusions from younger people. But this is very risky. Blood transfusions can carry the risk of blood-related diseases such as the Zika virus. Or back in the 1980s, HIV and hepatitis C transmission could easily happen. The results also don't last. This led some biohackers to take the real thing, GDF-11. GDF-11 is an injection. Biohackers buy it from experimental labs, and they reported that they turned back their biological age by a decade or more. But this is also risky because this peptide can cause serious palpitations. No one really knows the right dose. This peptide is currently not commercially available. It is sold under the radar but may be available to the public when more research becomes available.

Klotho

A promising protein that can make us live long is called klotho. This protein injection is also not commercially available to the public for now. Some people buy it on the black market. Klotho is a protein made in the kidneys. The discovery of klotho protein was also purely accidental. In Japan, a scientist worked on a mouse that had his gene for the klotho protein deleted and the mouse died prematurely of old age at the age of two months. Mice usually live two years. The scientist then worked on mice with elevated levels of the klotho protein, and these mice lived longer by 30 percent more, to three years of age. It appears that the klotho protein plays a huge role in longevity.

Some biohackers buy klotho protein from lab manufacturers. But no one knows the klotho dose in humans for longevity. Klotho injections also have some serious side effects such as palpitations.

High klotho levels have been linked to people with higher IQ and a longer lifespan. Klotho levels increase with exercise. Certain supplements can increase klotho naturally, such as activated charcoal, pterostilbene, gentian root extract, and probiotics.

In *The Ageless Revolution*, I have taken you for a ride from basic information on nutrition to the most futuristic treatments that are done overseas. I covered almost everything from A to Z. I covered what is affordable and what is cost prohibitive. I gave plenty of affordable alternatives. A whole new bright world is waiting for us. It's important to be cautious too. Some biohackers use futuristic therapies such as GDF-11 or klotho without knowing the long-term effects on longevity. With so many advances already here or in the pipeline, the future is bright. We are on the cusp of conquering aging.

A Patient's Story

Nancy was a fifty-five-year-old patient from Chicago who came to me looking for alternative medical therapies to help with her health problems. Nancy was overweight, at five feet two inches, she weighed 180 pounds, and her body mass index was thirty-four, which was very high. She also had high blood pressure, high cholesterol, and used a sleep apnea machine. Nancy was on several medications for her chronic health problems and followed a low-fat diet. She could not exercise due to severe knee pain related to her weight and had stopped working. She also suffered a mini stroke for which she was taking aspirin. With all these comorbidities, her future did not look bright. So after several consultations, she started on her ageless journey.

I placed her on the ageless diet, weight-loss peptides, and the right supplements. She also started on hyperbaric oxygen chamber sessions. One year later, Nancy was down to 130 pounds, and she was off her blood pressure and cholesterol medications. Her mind was sharp, and she no longer needed the sleep apnea machine after the dramatic weight loss.

Remember . . .

- Enhanced counterpulsation can be used for circulatory issues.
- Breathing oxygen while working out is already done by professional athletes.
- *Hyperbaric oxygen chamber* is too expensive and time-consuming for the average person. But if you have medical issues, try to get your insurance to cover it.
- You can already find Power Plates in many fancy gyms. It can help you build more muscle.
- Exosome treatment is in the preliminary stages for longevity but has already shown benefits for skin rejuvenation, hair growth, and arthritis.
- *Rapamycin* still needs more professional research, but it improves the way DNA is stored in cells. It renews the energy and strength of

dying DNA cells and encourages the growth of proteins that help DNA to stay intact and cells to form. It could be very promising.

- Gene and cell therapy are in the early stages for treating many diseases.

- The FDA does not allow the compounding of peptides in pharmacies.

- You can still find some doctors who have access to peptides.

- GDF-11 is a promising new longevity peptide. It is a futuristic peptide.

- Klotho protein is a promising anti-aging protein.

CHAPTER 22

Finding the Right Doctor

Medicines cure diseases
but only doctors can cure patients.
—Carl Jung

I hate to put you on the spot, but I have a few more questions for you. Are you up-to-date with your yearly physical? Are you up-to-date with your routine vaccines? There are countless excuses why you might be late. But if you aim to change your health, you need to flip your brain's switch on to turn your life around. You need to be up-to-date on the routine preventive medicine, healthy living, before you embark on this new innovative way to age. You need to change your genetic destiny. The good news: you have found it here in *The Ageless Revolution*.

Whatever your health situation, when you picked this book, I am glad that I was able to share this life-changing information with you. By reading this book, you've learned how to age in a different way.

You probably already take care of yourself by going to your doctor once a year and getting a physical. That's good. There, he or she will take your blood pressure, listen to your heart and lungs, check for hernias, and draw your blood to run routine tests for sugar, cholesterol, etc. But, today, the traditional physical exam is almost useless. It does not give us the information we most need to know to prevent chronic disease and improve health and longevity.

Your doctor may also order blood tests like a CBC (complete blood count), measuring the cells that are made of myeloid stem cells, which are plentiful and do not decline with age. So, again, this approach falls short. This test tells us nothing about the lymphoid stem cells' status, which declines as we age. Yes, the doctor may suggest screening for breast or colon cancer, but 70 percent of cancer goes unscreened. It is time for a revolution in health care.

We need a new direction, a revolutionary plan designed to take advantage of the medical advances available in the twenty-first century. Just like when the panel light in your car tells you something is wrong, we need similar ways to monitor and take immediate ownership of our health to fill the gap caused by the traditional medicine approach. This can include things like gadgets that check our glucose levels and our heart rates, just like apps on smart phones that can check your oxygen level and how much sleep you get. Or watches and apps that track how many steps you take in one day. Let's face it, we can often get more useful information from those gadgets than from any physical exam. So go to your iPhone app, or smartphone, and see which apps can help you in this new anti-aging journey.

Testing, Testing

You need the right doctor too. Doctors now also have tests to check your telomeres' length, your sex hormone levels, NAD levels, klotho levels, vitamin levels, and how much plaque you have in your arteries. Of course, there are also tests to check your biological age. You can even get a whole-body MRI to look at the body's organs. We have blood tests to check for over fifty types of cancer. We now have telemedicine so you can see your doctor from the comfort of your own home. But is your doctor aware of all these tests?

Be Proactive in Your Own Health Care

We have many new tools to aid us in our quest to be healthier and live longer, but most of the time, we aren't proactive. We only go to the doctor when we are sick. If we get a physical, sometimes we do not even follow up or act on the test results. How many of you are falling behind on your colonoscopy or abnormal test results that your doctor told you to follow up on?

Now that you understand the importance of a healthy diet, exercise, supplements, anti-aging medications, hormone replacement, and more, you need to find a partner to help you in your mission to prevent chronic diseases, stay young, and live your best life.

Finding the Right Doctor for You

Yes, many of the things that you have learned through the pages of *The Ageless Revolution* you can accomplish on your own. However, finding the right doctor who understands breakthroughs, anti-aging treatments including metformin, peptides, and bioidentical hormones, and all the topics I discussed in this book will be a big help.

Yes, you'll need to look for the right doctor. It's a bit like dating. You know it is tough out there, but you are still secretly hoping to find the right one, and you can.

The right doctor for you might be your primary care physician (PCP) or a functional medicine doctor, or have a different specialty, but he or she must be knowledgeable about new anti-aging treatments. Remember, you'll be entrusting that doctor with your health care and your life.

You might even need a few doctors, and that is perfectly okay. You might need a primary care doctor who gives you metformin, a gynecologist who can give you bioidentical hormones, and an orthopedic surgeon to inject PRP or exosomes in your knees if you have arthritis. You may need a dermatologist who can give you the latest laser skin treatment or exosomes after microneedling to renew your collagen. Unlike dating, this is not cheating.

Most importantly, you need to find the right professionals who are up-to-date on these advances.

Aging should not be about Botox, fillers, and facelifts. It should be a new model to fight aging at the cellular level. However, the reality is that your regular doctor may have a good education and good intentions, but he might not know all the information in this book. As doctors, we are not trained to treat aging on the cellular level, and only some of the recommendations in this book are standard medical advice. Much of what I've covered is new information that the medical community has yet to embrace.

So you'll really need to find a doctor who is open-minded and practices not only traditional medicine, but anti-aging, complementary, functional, or regenerative medicine. You need to be able to ask him or her questions about treatments you think may benefit you. For example, you might ask: "Have you heard about dihydroberberine? It improves sugar levels. Do you think it is the right supplement for me?" Or "I heard metformin is a longevity drug. Do you think I am a candidate for it based on my sugar level or my kidney function?" The most important thing is that he or she must be open-minded enough to tell you, "I will look it up." It is a patient who introduced me to grounding, and I looked it up after her joint pain was gone. I am perfectly okay to be a student at my age.

Depending on your needs, your doctor needs to be up-to-date or willing to learn about the progressive treatments that will best suit you.

Does Your Doctor Recognize the Ten Hallmarks of Aging?

Most importantly, he or she must recognize all the ten hallmarks of aging. This is a new arena, a new frontier that opens all the possibilities to conquer aging. He or she must be willing and able to prescribe and administer the new and increasingly expanding anti-aging treatments and therapy options as they become available. If he or she does not know, give him or her a copy of this book. Information is power.

How to Find the Right Doctor

You can find your new doctor through your insurance provider, word of mouth, social media, Vitals, or even Google, for starters.

Read online patient reviews that talk about a doctor's background, treatments provided, history with patients, and attitude. The doctor should have a willingness to really hear what you are saying, not talk down to you or in a manner so clinical that the information is hard to grasp.

Check the doctor's website. If he or she seems like a good fit, call. Keep in mind that you are allowed to call around to different offices and make preliminary appointments with different providers so you can get a sense of which one you like. This kind of doctor-shopping is common when expectant parents interview different pediatricians. There is no reason you cannot do the same to find your own doctor.

Before you make your appointment, ask the receptionist if the doctor prescribes peptides or bioidentical hormones. Do they offer NAD drips? Again, ask questions based on your specific medical needs. If you're satisfied with the information you gather and it feels right, make the appointment and see if he or she is a good fit for you.

Before your first appointment you'll need to be ready with a summary of your personal and family history, current prescriptions and dietary supplements, any allergies, and your lifestyle habits and environment. It makes things easy. Discuss your main concerns before the physical exam. Depending on your needs, complaints, and medical history, your doctor may request conventional lab tests or more advanced labs, imaging, or X-rays.

Often a general practitioner does not order any functional testing: saliva testing for sex hormones and cortisol, food sensitivity, BRAC genetic testing, gut health to see your microbiome, and a comprehensive cancer screening. You may need to see a functional health-care practitioner to get a more complete picture of your health. This is important because you need to know what your baseline is, meaning where you are at the start of treatment before test treatments or new approaches that may or may not work to bring you optimal health.

In order to get your needs met, the time you spend with the doctor on your first visit is an important way to establish a rapport. Trusting in your doctor and having a partnership/relationship have better outcomes. A partnership can mean having a doctor who can check in with patients monthly to see how they are improving and adjust the medical care as needed. This can lead to a better outcome in helping patients achieve better health. This is quite different from the way most conventional primary care doctors work.

Do not address all your concerns in one visit. Keep the issues limited to one or two most important things so that you and your doctor can handle the issues appropriately. Neither you nor the doctor should become overwhelmed by the number of concerns or information.

The Right Connection Is Essential

You must feel comfortable with your medical doctor. Be on the lookout for someone who makes eye contact and listens without interrupting you. It is about more than just pleasantries. Going to a doctor who is empathetic and can help you stay on top of your choices is essential.

Not only must he or she have the right medical knowledge and experience, but personality is a factor. You must like the doctor and feel comfortable on a personal level. It will not work if the doctor is knowledgeable but aloof or grouchy. Although the doctor's medical knowledge is more important, you may start skipping appointments until you just do not go.

You *can* find a doctor with both the right expertise and a pleasant personality. It is important in the long run. "Find somebody who is curious, who asks questions that let you know that you are being heard," says Sana Goldberg, a nurse and the author of *How to Be a Patient.*

Furthermore, research shows that having a PCP you feel comfortable with can be critical to your well-being. A 2005 paper by Johns Hopkins pediatrician Barbara Starfield found that robust relationships with PCPs help prevent illness and death and can help reduce racial and socioeconomic health disparities.

Your Primary Doctor Is Your First Anti-Aging Partner

Your PCP is your first point of contact in the health-care system, someone who knows the full you, not just your kidneys or your heart. The doctor is there to help prevent you from getting sick and guides you through a complicated network of hospitals and specialists if you do become ill.

Your PCP may be able to lead you to the right doctor who can work in complementary ways with him or her, or act as your main go-to doc. It is not so unusual anymore for a primary care doctor to also be well educated in functional medicine and practice both.

How to Talk to Your Doctor

Try to be as honest as you can with your doctor as you start and continue your relationship. If you have an issue, tell your doctor how it makes you feel and try to keep your feedback positive but very specific. "I love how you care for me, but it makes me feel dismissed when you look at the computer more than me and do not explain the next steps or the plan." Or "I am having a hard time understanding the plan. Can you use fewer medical terms?" There is nothing wrong with some constructive and positive feedback. I gave this book as a draft copy to several lay people to get their opinions to make sure I am clear, and I am not talking like a doctor. Their input was very constructive. I always appreciate positive feedback that makes me improve my medical care.

The Benefits of Functional Medicine

Functional medicine is spreading advances in medicine and focuses on whole body wellness, cellular aging, wellness, vitality, and healing rather than on disease. An illness is more likely to happen when there is a physiologic imbalance. A functional or integrative doctor will focus on balance at all levels, from cellular to lifestyle, to treat and prevent the root cause of illness. That doctor will provide you with specific guidelines.

Most patients are thrilled to have a personalized, individual treatment plan and sometimes specific, personalized prescriptions, as I have mentioned throughout this book. The right doctor guides and informs patients about their personal treatment options. An honest agreement on treatment leads to higher compliance and likelihood of success. He or she must be open-minded.

Why You May Want to Choose a Functional Medicine Doctor

Functional medicine, or treating the underlying problem, is becoming more popular because of the high rates of chronic diseases, the prohibitive cost of conventional medical care, and patients who spread the word of their improved health and lifestyle. Because of this, the scientific community is starting to conduct more research into the results and safety of various forms of complementary therapies. Some medical schools have started to include complementary disciplines in their curricula.

A paper published in the *Journal of the American Medical Association* in 2022 noted that 48 percent of mainstream doctors recommend complementary protocols to their patients, and 24 percent of doctors use some form of it themselves.

Get the Right Tests to Start

Once you decide you've found the right doctor, you can see if anti-aging tests including NAD levels, telomere length, klotho levels, and uric acid are available. In general, to start, I suggest you ask your doctor to run these five blood tests first. Those tests can give an idea about your health, so you can take action before going to the next level.

Lipoprotein(a)

One in five Americans lives with high lipoprotein(a). Often this fact means suffering a sudden heart attack like what happened to Bob Harper, from *The Biggest Loser,* at age fifty-two. This test checks for your LPA genotype because certain LPA gene expressions are associated with increased risk for blood vessel diseases, stroke, and heart attack. If this one time test indicates an increased risk, your health-care provider might suggest losing weight, exercise, niacin, or taking a medication like metformin. There is a new drug that should be out soon called Muvalapin. Desirable levels should be below 30 mg/dl.

APOE Gene

APOE gene is one of the most powerful predictors of whether you have a predisposition to develop Alzheimer's disease. Some doctors do not want to run that test for cost, but I truly believe the risks for Alzheimer's disease can be minimized with the right lifestyle choices. Exercising, intermittent fasting, lowering alcohol consumption, quitting smoking, and getting enough sleep have been linked to lower the Alzheimer's risk—even in people with high genetic risk.

ApoB

An ApoB test measures ApoB levels, the main protein found in the low-density lipoproteins (LDL), which is more predictive of cardiovascular diseases than simply LDL. LDL is the bad cholesterol that has the potential to damage your heart and arteries in high concentrations. ApoB should be completed annually. Although this test is usually not covered by insurance, don't let your health-care provider persuade you not to do it for the cost; it is about twenty dollars. If your levels are high, your doctor may suggest avoiding tobacco and exercising more. Desirable levels should be 65 to 80 mg/dL.

Hemoglobin A1c (HbA1c)

HbA1c measures your average blood sugar level over the previous three months and is commonly used to diagnose and manage diabetes and prediabetes. The HbA1c test can help diabetics maintain optimal glucose or can tell you if you are prediabetic. Levels should be less than 5.6.

Gamma-Glutamyl Transpeptidase (GGT)

Gamma-glutamyl transferase (GGT) is an enzyme primarily produced by the liver and is known as a sensitive indicator of liver and biliary disease and damage. Elevated GGT is associated with an increased risk of many conditions, including cardiovascular disease, stroke, metabolic syndrome, insulin resistance, diabetes, obesity, hypertension, fatty liver, and all-cause mortality. If it is high, you need to address your lifestyle such as cutting down on alcohol and fructose. GGT levels should be below 30 IU/L.

Ways to Reduce Costs on *The Ageless Revolution*

You need to take care of yourself by eating right and exercising. Anything else you do after reading this book is extra and a bonus. Buy taurine; it is cheap. Look for Power Plate at your gym, use the gym sauna, do a cold plunge at home. If you decide to pursue anti-aging at a functional doctor, call to see if the doctor takes your insurance. Bioidentical hormones or testosterone should be covered by your insurance. Get the brands covered by your plan from a local pharmacy. Medical groups and insurance concerns often make money by spending no more than fifteen minutes with each patient. Given this fact, health care in the twenty-first century is more like the eighteenth century. So, once you find the right doctor who takes your insurance, be mindful of time and meet with a doctor several times to cover all your concerns. Be smart, use your money wisely.

Doctors Need to Lead the Way in Anti-Aging

Biohackers, like athletes, are becoming more and more knowledgeable and are sharing these advances in medicine treatments like bioidentical hormone replacement, peptides, exosome treatments, cryotherapy, and all the other health and anti-aging treatments on Instagram and TikTok. But I think that it's the doctors who should start the revolution and bring innovative information to the masses, not the other way around. However, I am glad many of my young patients are aware of the benefits of intermittent fasting, cryotherapy, and peptides. Only when doctors start treating aging as a disease can an ageless society happen.

When It's Time to Break Up with Your Doctor

If you tried a new doctor but still don't feel like it's the right fit or you're not being heard, it may be time to break up. It is always okay to go to another doctor who understands new treatments. When you meet a new potential doctor, feel free to tell him or her what was not working with your old one. It will ensure starting off on the right foot. It might be frustrating to start your search again, but it is worth it. It is your life.

Whether you are in the process of finding a new doctor or not, you still need to take care of your blood pressure, sugar levels, and specific ongoing illnesses with your traditional doctor. Again, what you've read here is in addition to, not a substitute for, your standard medical care, including vaccines, colonoscopy, mammograms, and other tests and procedures. However, following *The Ageless Revolution* will improve your health and longevity even more. My goal is to make your future as bright as possible!

A Patient's Story

Cyndi's story will show you what a difference healthy lifestyle changes can make. Cyndi was fifty-five, 5 feet 2 inches, and 200 pounds when she first came to see me. She followed a low-fat diet but could not stick to it all the time as she was always hungry. She had high blood pressure, high cholesterol, type 2 diabetes, arthritis, and sleep apnea, and her blood work had some kidney impairment. Her orthopedist suggested a bilateral knee replacement for her arthritis. She took tons of medications including synthetic hormones prescribed by her gynecologist. Her copays were close to $15,000 a year. She was off work for a few weeks and wanted to go on long-term disability. I had three visits in one month with Cyndi, during which we covered everything from diet to medications. With a new diet, the right supplements, and bioidentical hormones she was on the right track. Within three months, Cyndi lost twenty pounds. Within fourteen months, she was down to 140 pounds, her sugar was normal, her cholesterol improved, and her kidney functions normalized. Her knee pain was gone since she took all the weight off, and she no longer needed a knee replacement. She was back at her job as an account executive in a big financial firm. She now leads a vibrant and healthy life.

Remember . . .

- Find a doctor who can become your primary care physician, understands functional medicine and the ten hallmarks of aging, and can prescribe and administer the new treatments in this book.

- Shop around for a doctor. Use word of mouth, the Internet, your insurance provider, and read reviews. Call doctors' offices and ask what services and procedures are offered before making an appointment.

- If you realize at any time that you are not happy with your individual treatment plan, or the doctor him- or herself, it is okay to find someone else.

PART VI

Embrace
the Ageless Life

CHAPTER 23

Staying the Course

Committing to a lifetime of wellness is not a luxury—it's a necessity. You'll never have enough time; you have to make the time.
—**Oprah Winfrey**

In this book, we discovered the secrets of longevity from around the world as we delved into the fascinating world of centenarians of the Blue Zones. We went into the science behind their long lifespans. The discovery of the ten hallmarks of aging were a game changer. Scientists continue to look into plants, foods, and medications that can alter our genes. I explored how everything worked and how it impacts those ten hallmarks. The solutions were there, and I know you may feel a little overwhelmed with all this information. That's not the goal now that we have the defenses. If there was a cure for a terminal illness, would you take it? I don't know of anyone who would not sign up. It must be the same for aging, a terminal illness with a fatal end. Many of the cures are natural. So let's start the treatment.

When starting *The Ageless Revolution,* it is important to take a basic, slow, and steady approach. For inspiration, look to the people who live in the five Blue Zones. They have longevity. They eat right and exercise. They don't need any of the treatments, supplements or medications, or science discussed here. But in most of the Western world we do need to make conscious and conscientious changes to improve our health. I believe *The Ageless Revolution* fills that gap. It tells where we went wrong. It tells us how we can change course. Again, I want everyone to be a participant, not just the rich who already have access to this information. *The Ageless Revolution* is for the masses, the forgotten men and women in our broken health-care system.

My Learning Curve

I'm a lifelong learner. My training did not stop after medical school. I became a doctor to make people's lives healthier and help them live longer and better. This can only happen through continuous learning. Armed with this information, extending the lifespan of my patients and keeping them healthy for life with this new knowledge are my top priority. I no longer want to put Band-Aids on diseases; I want real change in health care. I want you to change direction too. Do it slowly like me.

If I reflect on my life, I will say I had a good life if it all ends today. I had my ups and downs, but I've accomplished everything I set out to do. Still, my health was always on the back burner. My career, my patients always took priority. My health should have always been my top priority in order for me to take care of others, but it wasn't. In my thirties I was very stressed, my blood pressure was high, I had prediabetes, and I was overweight. I knew that I had to change my perspective on life, and I did. I improved my health with little changes and efforts. Life is meant to be enjoyed. It's very short no matter how long we stay in this world. I did it in stages.

As I approach my sixth decade on earth, I look at myself now—I am happy and calm, have life's wisdom, and I am healthy. My blood pressure has normalized, my prediabetes is gone, and I sleep well. My energy level is very good, and I run three miles three times a week. I look at myself in the mirror, I am fitter than ever, I have no apparent skin damage or wrinkles. My mind is sharp, and I recollect things quickly like a teenager. Some people question my age because of my energy and appearance. I do not see myself at my chronological age at all. My efforts are turning my dream into a reality. I reflect on my book title, and say gee, I am really becoming ageless. You too can turn your health around with *The Ageless Revolution.*

As you continue your life's journey, I urge you to take control of your health. Have an unconventional outlook to manage your age versus accepting it. Evolution-wise you are a tiny speck on a floating rock with 8 billion other people on it. No one cares about your health but you. We are all destined to get sick, old, and die. But you can use this truth to fuel your efforts to be healthier and live longer. Roll up your sleeves and consider your health as a job—your main job. Take your health seriously. Remove the roadblocks from your mind and life. Transform your health by conquering your cells. A new outlook means a new future. Think of this book as a road map to a new beginning, a revolution to a new you.

Getting Started on *The Ageless Revolution*

You've learned all about the ten hallmarks of aging in this book and the ways to target each of them with a variety of programs, strategies, and treatments including diet, exercise, lifestyle, and more advanced approaches. I brought you longevity secrets from all over the world from the people who have lived the longest.

This may feel overwhelming. So don't try to follow everything I recommend; instead, start slowly and, most importantly, act. To accomplish your a*geless* goals, you must have a three-point strategy.

First, depending on your needs, set your own goal, next plan, then act. Maybe if you are overweight, your first goal would be to lose weight. Plan it, then act on it. It is also important to get rid of all negative things you do before you start all the positive things I recommend. It would be good to find the right doctor who can help you with your next steps with hormones and regenerative medicine. No rush. Read *The Ageless Revolution* again. Allow yourself to digest all the information in this book. I want you to understand science and be inspired and dedicated.

Simple Changes Are Life-Changing

Where do you start? Write down all the negative things you do. Give yourself a negative score for each bad thing you do. It is important to reach zero. Drinking too much? Cut down or stop. Smoking? Stop. Now that you went from a score of minus two to zero, start the positives. Eating right has the most impact on longevity. It can add fourteen years to your life. Going to bed early can make you live three years longer. Floss daily, and this can add three to five years as you get rid of the bad bacteria in your mouth. Having more sex can add eight years. All this is doable and will be easy to implement in the first few weeks. Next, intermittent fasting should be next on your to-do list. It can probably add nine years to your life. Skip breakfast two days a week. Do it on weekends. Always eat dinner early. Do not eat later than 5 or 6 PM. This could be a little challenging initially, but it is certainly doable. Next, start walking. Walking thirty minutes a day can make you live 2.2 years longer. Eventually, you can up your exercise routine. Eventually add strength training. It can add another 1.8 years to your life. If you are fit and healthy, try HIIT. Next on your list should be the supplements. Start with fish oil and taurine. Try to add twenty minutes to your gym routine so that you can spend some time in the steam room. Finally, find a doctor who can help you with medications. The cumulative effect of all these measures will easily add twenty-plus years. I do not think the sky's the limit, but I guess the limit has been extended beyond the norm. Do not make excuses. An extra two to three hours a week to take better care of your body will have a great impact on your longevity.

The New Way to Age Is Already Here

The Ageless Revolution is indeed comprehensive. It is a lot of information to digest, not only for the layperson, but for doctors as well. But I feel that it's the minimal amount of information you need to change your destiny. I made it to the point and straightforward.

For most people, aging is a fact of life: We must accept it; it is natural! I say, absolutely not! When your expensive car gets old and needs engine oil, do you say, "My car is old," and leave it to die, or do you go to fix it and add oil? Implementing *The Ageless Revolution* is a way to fix and maintain your body. Take advantage of it, and you can kick the can far, far down the road. Missing NAD? Replace it. Low in vitamin D? Take it. Missing sex hormones? Replenish them.

Often, though, in these days of self-love (nothing wrong with that), we are told to embrace everything, including aging. It is okay now to be overweight and do nothing about it. It is okay to get three old-age-related diseases by the time we are fifty or sixty years old, and say it is part of getting old. Even doctors tell us aging is okay. They tell menopausal women who are suffering, "Your hormones are normal! Take Valium or Prozac."

We don't need to accept this antiquated approach when we have so many medical advances and measures that are here and can make a great impact. Anti-aging medications and hormones are just the beginning of this revolution.

My Journey to *The Ageless Revolution* Was a Very Long Road

It was not until I was in my fifties that I had my own health revolution. My career, life, and misinformation derailed me. Looking after my health was supposed to be the most important thing in life, but I did not. I am sure many of you are in the same boat, so the time to do *The Ageless Revolution* is now.

You never know where life lessons are going to come from. Sometimes, it's an event that makes you realize you must change everything. You need to act and take your health seriously. For me, the lesson came in my late thirties when I had nonstop tremors and I thought I had Parkinson's disease. It was stress, as I've mentioned before. Regardless, the negative became a positive, and I decided to take care of my health and begin my own anti-aging journey.

At one time, I was like you. In the past, I did nothing to revive and invigorate my body and mind. In fact, I did tons of bad and harmful things to my body. I followed a low-fat diet. I ate frozen "healthy" dinners to lose weight. I ate margarine. I thought nuts were bad. I ate every three hours, thinking it would keep me thin and my metabolism going. I stayed up late watching TV most nights. It is everything I advocate against now. In no time, I became overweight. I blindly followed outdated guidelines from the medical establishment and didn't use my intelligence. In fact, most of these guidelines and measures accelerated my aging versus targeted the ten hallmarks of aging.

It was not until I was in my early forties, and I retrained in functional medicine, that I started to clean my diet. This did not happen until I cleared my mind of all the misinformation. My philosophy on disease, what I teach patients, and what I write in columns had to change. This resulted in my writing *The Perfect 10 Diet* to make a difference in people's lives.

Going against the herd is not an easy thing to do. But I had to be 100 percent correct before going on national TV correcting outdated and antiquated medical establishment guidelines. I had to explain that some were just plain wrong. I was against low-fat, low-carb, and keto diets. I advocated for a balanced diet with natural food with normal amounts of fats, not massive amounts of fats like both low-carb and keto! On television shows, radio, and in the media, I explained that saturated fats are not bad; they are good.

I was a guest on *Fox and Friends,* and they questioned how palm oil, a saturated fat, can be good when medical recommendations say it is a bad fat. I told them, "These are old guidelines." I don't want to be labeled a rebel or called crazy; I just want to help people.

The latest research is on my side. But that is not what the mainstream establishment will tell you. By following the herd, we are not exploring the new frontiers and the new discoveries out there. I did enormous damage to my health by following bad recommendations. So, if you are younger and reading this book, you are indeed lucky. You are on your way to adding twenty to twenty-five years of longevity to your life.

One day while in line at Starbucks, I had a revelation. I was the only one in line asking the barista for a full-fat turmeric latte. Not low-fat or skim milk. I wanted to tell the l other people in the line, "Don't order that low-fat frappuccino." Instead, I'm trying to reach a wider audience with this book and change what people think is healthy.

My Health and Longevity Routine Today

Now, I do intermittent fasting a few days a month. I eat organic foods. I take supplements and use the sauna at the gym. I do HIIT even though it is intense and not particularly enjoyable, but I know it is good for me. At the gym, I use the Power Plate and the steam sauna. I bought a small red light therapy unit for home use. I use it two to three times on weekends and I find it relaxing. I go for cryotherapy whenever I have the time. I go to the dermatologist to get a microneedling or a laser treatment to rejuvenate my skin once or twice a year. I want to be as healthy as I can for myself and my patients. I certainly don't do everything in this book. I wish I had the time to do hyperbaric oxygen, but I am aware of all the anti-aging options.

Whatever your age is now, we are all in the same boat. It is never too late to start. Keep a positive attitude. Do not think of all these new tasks as obstacles; they are possibilities. Possibilities for a healthier life, a lifespan of prosperity, and more time for you to be on this earth with your friends, family, and loved ones. You can't put a price on that. Look at each day as a new beginning in your journey to live a longer and healthier life. You may do the wrong thing one day, or one week, or on a vacation, and it is perfectly okay. You are only human. I am not perfect, either. Just keep your eyes on the big goal, and get back on track.

Here Are the Most Important Things to Remember as You Embark on Your Ageless Journey

Rid Yourself of Bad Habits. I cannot stress this enough. Unhealthy habits will sabotage any of your efforts to be healthy and stay healthy. Nothing in this book will work if you have unhealthy habits. Unhealthy habits alter your epigenome in the wrong way.

Eat Clean. Fresh vegetables and low-sugar fruits are your friends. Stay away from low-fat products with added sugar, processed foods, and fad diets that interfere with your health. Eliminate—or significantly reduce—your daily intake of sugar. Sugar is bad, but other chemicals in low-carb products and nitrites are not good for you either. Avoid low-carb or keto diets. These diets may give you the weight loss you desire, but they are not good for longevity. In fact, they may shorten your life. Again, what matters is the inside, not the outside. Choose the superfoods and spices I've recommended to rev up and help heal your body. Go organic for the food choices if you can, and buy wild food from online stores. Have a variety of teas at your house.

Try Intermittent Fasting. Remember, there is solid logic in when to eat or not to eat. Try one of the fasts I recommended. It is so easy to skip a meal.

Exercise Your Body and Mind Regularly. Incorporate exercise in your daily life with simple tasks. Once a week is a safe way to start; eventually, try to exercise at least three times a week or more. Find what you like to do. Maybe it is tennis, jogging, or lifting weights. It is all good. It does not have to be HIIT—whatever gets you moving will be okay. Get the circulation going to your brain and muscles. Strengthen your bones. Give your brain a workout too by eating right and learning new words every day or learning a new language. French or Italian—whatever appeals to you to challenge your brain.

Take the Right Supplements. Start with three to four supplements before you add more. Supplements can give you a boost and help promote longevity.

Buy them from reputable vitamin stores or my website: www.theAgelessRev-olution.com. If you can't afford the supplements that affect cell age, change your lifestyle. Again, many centenarians in the five Blue Zones made it to one hundred years without taking a single supplement. You can do it too.

Utilize Good Stress. You've learned about good or hormetic stress. Try one or two of the new things I have told you about. Choose a way to activate hermetic stress that appeals to you and invigorates your body. Use the sauna at your gym after your workouts more often. Occasionally take a cold bath. A cool plunge pool is available in many gyms. You can even do it in your own bathtub. Use the cryotherapy chamber at a spa if you can afford it. Try red light therapy. All are affordable options. You deserve to live a full, rich life.

Find a Functional Medicine Doctor to Take The Ageless Revolution to the Next Level. Functional medicine is growing in respect, demand, and availability. Most primary care physicians are traditional in their approach. They treat an ailment or disease after it shows up. Functional doctors com-bine their traditional studies with a newer approach: cellular aging. These doctors treat the entire body as a whole and are concerned with keeping you healthy to avoid illness in the first place. You want this kind of doctor.

Try Anti-Aging Beauty Treatments. Today enhancements for skin anti-aging should not be about Botox and fillers at your dermatologist, but cellular aging as well. Stem cells, exosomes, and the right anti-aging supple-ments will help you reverse your skin's biological age. Find a dermatologist that uses these new and innovative treatments like microneedling. You do not have to do expensive laser treatments at your cosmetic dermatologist to have beautiful skin. You can do a regular skin routine right from your own home.

Do Not Get Derailed. I cannot emphasize this enough. Stay on track. It is easy to get unintentionally derailed by well-meaning family, friends, and coworkers who have different ideas and approaches to how to live and be healthy. A night of partying and drinking or drugs may be living life for them, but for you, it is nothing but a sabotage to your life.

Lifestyle changes like moving, traveling, starting a new relationship or ending one, or a holiday celebration can disrupt eating, sleeping, and activity routines. Life happens. Recognize what is going on and get back on track right away. Keep a positive attitude, and your eyes on the goal—an ageless life—and you will get through any obstacle.

I finish this chapter by sharing a story to emphasize the fact that the time to look after yourself is right now. Waiting is a losing game. In 1928, Alexander Fleming discovered penicillin, and by the 1940s this antibiotic became the greatest advance in therapeutic medicine to date. Before antibiotics, people died of pneumonia, syphilis, meningitis, and tuberculosis. In the 1930s, the average lifespan was 58.5 years. Antibiotics were a game changer. Antibiotics increase lifespans by as much as twenty years. Fleming was a genius scientist, but he was not a great communicator. It took fourteen more years for penicillin to be commercialized after his discovery. In those fourteen years, millions of people who could have been saved by penicillin's discovery died unnecessarily from various infections. Ten years ago, the ten hallmarks of aging were discovered, yet no one is talking about them! Why is that? No one has complied with all the weapons against them. I hope I was a great communicator. I made it as simple as I can. My goal with *The Ageless Revolution* is to bring this information to as many people as possible. There is a solution for our many health issues. Take advantage of the information and change your life. Some may think this book is futuristic, but the future is already here. Let us not stay in the dark. It is time to live your best life now.

Remember . . .

- Start slow. Do not start everything on *The Ageless Revolution* all at once.
- Get rid of unhealthy habits—smoking, drugs, excess alcohol, too much food. You know them all. Reduce stress.
- Eat clean. Go organic with produce and whatever else is possible.

- Read labels on meat, eggs, milk, and poultry, and cut out sugar! Try to eat some wild food. Buy it from online retailers.

- Exercise. Start with a fifteen-minute walk and build from there. Do some HIIT if you are fit enough.

- Take appropriate supplements that are geared to your current physical health and needs.

- Utilize good stress. Explore new treatments that you can afford, or for the first time, use some at-home methods like ice-cube baths or hot saunas.

- Fasting helps you feel good physically and mentally. You have a choice of three different ones in this book.

- Find a doctor who practices functional, regenerative, and complementary medicine.

CHAPTER 24

Becoming Ageless Through a Purpose

The meaning of life is to find your gift.
The purpose of life is to give it away.
—**Pablo Picasso**

What do you want to accomplish in your life? What legacy do you want to leave? What is your life's purpose? Is your goal to live longer for your family and to see your grandchildren grow? Or is it something bigger—your community! It doesn't matter whether your purpose is big or small; the most important thing is to have a purpose.

Getting older is not the end of the road; it could be a new beginning. For the first time in history, many men and women continue to flourish and work past retirement age. Dolly Parton, who is in her late seventies, wants to sing for the rest of her life. Bruce Springsteen continues to tour in his seventies. Martha Stewart made it on the cover of *Sports Illustrated* at age eighty-one wearing a bathing suit. Lily Tomlin and Jane Fonda continue to make movies in their late eighties. Betty White continued to work until she died at the age of ninety-nine. A great life at an older age can be just the beginning for you.

By reading this book, you are already embracing the challenge to practice a multitude of ways to live longer with vibrant health and a radiant vitality. You are discovering things about yourself and your body, right down to the cellular level.

You are on track to living a longer and healthier life. What are you going to do with those added years? What are you doing now to not only live longer but also to be happier?

Life is precious and we need to enjoy the gift we were given when we came into this world. Negative attitudes are bad for brain health. We all need something to live for, a sense of meaning in our lives, a reason to get out of bed in the morning, and a reason to smile. If you have no purpose, your brain will tell your organs to shut down.

Without a purpose, it is easy to become depressed as you feel unfulfilled, aimless, and hopeless. Your immune system will be compromised. Purpose can be defined as a self-organizing life aim that stimulates goals. Or more simply, purpose means finding meaning in daily experiences, having reachable goals, and having a sense that life is important and worth living. It is about what you think is most valuable to you—community, achievement, relationships, spirituality, kindness. There is not a specific definition for any one person.

The Purpose and Happiness Cycle

Purpose brings you happiness, and happiness contributes to good health. Good health can provide a long life. Longer life helps grow purpose. It's a beautiful cycle. Withdrawing from community and isolating yourself can lead to heart disease, type 2 diabetes, dementia, and even suicide. You will age prematurely and have a shorter lifespan. Believe it or not, loneliness can truly be much worse than smoking; it will shorten your life. Historically, purpose and meaning came naturally. Survival depended on it. People joined together to find food and shelter, safety in numbers, and mutual support, and to tackle projects too big for one person alone. Communities were formed, grew, and multiplied.

Community is built on a network of family, friends, and strangers—let us say newcomers—who share common goals. Our family is our first community. There needs to be mutual support in caring for one another with unconditional love and acceptance. Shared experiences make connections and appreciation for one another stronger. Quality leisure time together can help manage stress. Nurturing relationships can also give us purpose.

However, today we are more connected on the Internet than in real life! We are separated from our families and friends by computers, tablets, and cell phones. Some of us are glued to social media and are totally separated from the real world. Virtual reality will only make this worse.

We've forgotten what it means to be connected and present in the moment or how to enjoy the relationships we have with one another. Having dinner with friends who are glued to social media apps while eating is not only impolite but also not enjoyable. They're present physically but totally absent mentally, and it sends a message that your time is not as valuable as the "likes" they are going to get from the picture of the food they feel obligated to share. It's time to go on a digital diet. Life is too short to waste time online. Be present in the moment, be present in life.

People in the Blue Zones often live to one hundred years of age or more. In Okinawa, a "reason for being" is a concept important to all. It is called ikigai. In Costa Rica, it is called the "plan de vida." Both include strong ties to family and community. Having meaning and a purpose, along with a thoughtful diet that keeps you healthy, contributes to your longevity.

There are many great reasons to have purpose in your life. People with supportive family and friends, or meaningful, rewarding work, can manage pain and anxiety better, catch fewer colds, report being more satisfied with their overall health, and often live longer.

Having Purpose Extends Your Lifespan

Celeste Leigh Pearce, associate professor in the department of epidemiology at the University of Michigan, showed the association between life purpose and health outcomes. Pearce admitted that she was skeptical about life's purpose when she and some colleagues explored the topic using data from the Health and Retirement Study, a national study of people ages fifty and older. The earliest participants were enrolled in the study in 1992 and had an average age of 68.6 years and were asked to complete a questionnaire about their life purpose. Researchers looked at causes of death in the group between 2006 and 2010. Variables including demographics, marital status, race, education level, health, and lifestyle choices like smoking and drinking were considered.

Data revealed that the more strongly the participants felt they had a purpose in life, the lower the risk of dying. A person lacking purpose is very likely to be less active, and therefore, less healthy. Low scorers were 2.43 times more likely to die from heart, circulatory, digestive, and blood conditions compared to participants with the highest scores. Other studies found that low life purpose scores are associated with higher levels of inflammatory markers and stress hormones, and the shortening of telomeres is associated with aging, cancer, and death.

More studies from Rush University, University of Michigan, University of Minnesota, and the NeuroGrow Brain Fitness Center also indicate that having a purpose in life has powerful beneficial effects on your brain and body. It can lower the risks of Alzheimer's disease and stroke. It can also help stroke patients recover their cognitive functions, and generally reduce cognitive decline by 50 percent.

Having purpose also protects the hippocampus, which is important for storing memories, learning, and navigation, from atrophy. Amazingly, having a life purpose has been associated with an increase in its size. A healthy hippocampus also reduces the odds of developing sleep disturbances, lowers the risk of mortality because of cardiovascular health, reduces overall inflammation, and leads to less chance of chronic diseases, better ability to deal with stress, and lower odds of impairments in daily living and mobility disabilities.

Purpose can guide life decisions, influence behavior, shape goals, offer a sense of direction, and create meaning. It is our inner compass. We can grow older in a healthy way and be inspired by the things we do.

However, even the most active and purposeful people can go offtrack. The illness or death of a spouse or other loved one, an unhealthy relationship, divorce, tragedy, and disappointment can feel overwhelming. I got derailed a few years ago when I lost my dad. Over time, I realized I had to get back on track, not only for myself, but for my patients. My purpose in life is bigger than my individuality. Maybe my purpose in life is to reach people beyond the boundaries of my office and to make a difference.

Purpose in life and your job or career may not be the same thing. Yet retirement, and the year immediately following, is a vulnerable time. For some, the end of a career means the end of purpose in life. Leaving your occupation behind can certainly affect health and well-being. Even people who have been able to retire early, say at age fifty-five, can be more vulnerable. So what can you do to find life's purpose and keep your life fulfilling, healthy, and long?

Your Purpose: Be the Best New Version of Yourself

Many of you may know of Tony Robbins, an author, life coach, motivational speaker, and philanthropist. Like myself, he is interested in the innovations of biohacking. He acknowledges that the best place to start biohacking is with diet, exercise, and mindfulness exercises. He advocates and reportedly uses cryotherapy, red light therapy, intermittent fasting, and other new techniques I told you about.

Change Your Brain Activity

Robbins points out that brain activity can be measured in a wavelike pattern and determines if you feel alert, sleepy, relaxed, or stressed. Music is a form of biohacking that uses beats and tones to synchronize with your brain waves and induce a meditative, relaxed state. Movie soundtracks are a good example. You can sit back in a recliner and let your mind drift, or bop to the beat of your favorite music while you make a meal if you want to wake your brain.

You can also learn a new language. Solve crosswords. Learn to play the piano. Include exercise in your life to have strong muscles and bones.

Robbins also stands by traditional habits like yoga and meditation as forms of biohacking to calm his mind and open it to new ideas and creativity. This may also help you reach deep into your being to find purpose. Start with a meditation ritual, or daily uplifting affirmations, to set a positive tone for your day.

Take Stock of Your Goals, Strengths, and Talents

You can start off by writing down your goals in life. It is the opposite of a bucket list. This can help you gain perspective on where you are and where you are going next in the added years. Recognize your strengths and talents. Write down what you are good at. Make time for your emotional and mental self-care as I hope you have done for your body and mind while using the knowledge you have found reading this book.

Read and Feed Your Mind

Nonfiction books help us make sense of the world but there is something to be said for a good novel. Read fiction too. It can connect you with people across time, place, and culture. It can improve your empathy and critical and creative thinking. Put yourself in the character's shoes, and see where it takes you.

Spend Time in Nature

Spend time in nature, and experience awe. Feeling awe helps us realize a connection to something bigger—yet part of ourselves. The poet Rumi reminds us: "You are not a drop in the ocean. You are the entire ocean in a drop." What this means is that to make peace with and respect the individuality of others, we have to accept and make peace with our own individuality.

Surround Yourself with Good People

Surround yourself with people who give meaning to your life, people who are positive, and who lift you up. They will inspire you to discover your unique purpose. Do not be afraid to ask trusted friends for feedback. Ask your friends what they value about you and what is your best quality and do the same for them.

Try a New Hobby

Try a new hobby or take a class about something you have always thought about but did not have the time to explore. Libraries and community schools offer a wealth of interesting, low-cost classes. You can discover talents you did not realize you had or hone the skills you already have.

Adopt a Pet

So many animals need good homes. You can do good for them and also do good for yourself. Having a pet can help you set daily routines, get exercise, and meet people either in your neighborhood or at the dog park. It can improve your physical, mental, and emotional health, and encourage social interaction. Studies show that pet owners are more likely to volunteer and support charities. It is important to take steps that affect and improve your purpose. Growing up, I never thought of having a pet. Now, I am a huge animal lover and love to contribute to animal charities. They bring me so much joy.

Volunteer

Volunteering can get you out of the house and help you focus on the needs of others rather than your own worries, aches, and pains. You can donate your time versus money. It helps you make new friends and develop a support system, and protects you from depression. You can find people with shared interests and have some fun. Volunteering counteracts stress, anger, and anxiety and builds a sense of accomplishment and overall well-being.

Researchers found by measuring brain activity and hormones that being helpful to others stimulates your own pleasure. Humans are hardwired to give to others. So the more you give, the happier you feel. The more connected to the community you are, the more purpose in life you experience. And you see here how much that boosts health and longevity.

Discover the Benefits of Sex

On a very personal level, a satisfying sex life goes a long way to longevity and purpose. If you can, sex should be part of your life, so rekindle intimacy with your spouse or partner. Studies show that sex is extremely beneficial to our health. It activates a variety of neurotransmitters that affect not only our brains but several other organs in our bodies.

The benefits of sex include:

- Lower blood pressure
- Immediate natural pain relief
- Lower risk for heart disease
- Lengthened telomeres
- Better immune system
- Improved sleep
- Increased libido
- Reduced physical and emotional stress
- Less depression and anxiety
- Improved skin

A good sex life can add years to your life. Your age doesn't matter. Older adults who want to stay sexually active have a multitude of aids to get them started. Movies, erotic literature, toys, role-playing . . . exploring things you have not done before can be quite arousing. For partners that can no longer perform because of disability or choose not to have sex, intimacy can be achieved by a steady habit of caring touches, holding hands, and being attentive to others' emotional needs. If you don't have a partner, why are you single? It is time to date again.

Practicing safe sex protects you from a variety of sexually transmitted diseases and unplanned pregnancies. It also sparks greater self-esteem, which contributes to being socially involved and more interested in pursuing your purpose in life.

Practice Gratitude

Gratitude is tied to well-being, so count your blessings. Literally take the time to keep a little gratitude journal. As Robbins and others have suggested, write down three to five things you are grateful for having in your life. Add the things that surprised you, and made you laugh, then do it daily, morning or night. Write a letter to someone who helped you at a particular time in your life. Look to people you admire, friends who do good. Pay wholehearted attention to mundane experiences—details you usually gloss over—and really listen to what someone is saying.

In the spring of 2023, I was invited to the Susan G. Komen charity's luncheon in New York City by their CEO, Mrs. Paula Schneider, to share her table. I was extremely moved by the generosity of the Susan G. Komen organization for women who have breast cancer. Just like Covid-19 killed more Americans than other Western nations, breast cancer affects women in the United States at much higher rates. It is also killing more minorities and women of color at a 40 percent higher rate. I was intensely moved by the personal survival stories. I realized how blessed I have been in my life despite all the ups and downs.

After writing this book, I decided to give the profits of *The Ageless Revolu tion* to help. For me, my revolution goal changed from making everyone live their best life with this book to making a difference for everybody on a humanitarian basis. I want to make a huge impact. I want to make life better for everyone. So join me in my journey, and let's make some noise. Share your ageless journey and *The Ageless Revolution* book on your Instagram, TikTok, and Facebook page. Let's go viral. I can't change the world alone, but together we all can. We can all make a difference and make the world healthier and a better place for the less fortunate. Give this book to your doctor too so he or she can learn about the new anti-aging advances. The revolution should be everywhere because a new beginning in health care has to start. We can no longer continue this disease-care path.

The Ageless Revolution has been a story of passion to change people's lives by getting the word out. It was a burning desire to change our health in the United States after the Covid-19 pandemic. When I was child, my goal in life was to be a physician. I never thought I would become an author. I never thought I could become a leader to give people information beyond my office.

I realize now that my purpose in life is much bigger than what I initially planned or envisioned. Finding and honoring your purpose is the foundation of a well-rounded, long life lived with robust vitality, happiness, and good health. A purpose in life makes you ageless. I know you are well on your way.

Remember . . .

- Write an honest list of your *strengths and talents.* If you need help on this one, talk to a trusted friend.

- Make a list of your *goals.* Yes, it is like a bucket list—but to start a new life or a new beginning.

- *Do something new.* Spend time in nature or read a book and notice how characters share or hold opposite views and goals from your own.

- *Volunteer* for an organization that is meaningful to you. You will discover how helping others will give you a sense of satisfaction.

- *Avoid negative people* and surround yourself with those who have a positive attitude.

- *Pay attention* to people when you talk to them. Look them in the eyes and really listen to what they are saying.

- *Have sex more often.* It delivers immediate benefits and encourages intimacy.

- *Adopt a pet.* Having one will give you the satisfaction of caring for another living creature who gives you unconditional love.

- *Profess gratitude.* As you wake up or go to sleep each day—or both—pick three things that make you feel grateful: a call from a friend, your renewed health, a bird on the windowsill—anything that makes you smile counts.

- *Show appreciation.* Write a note or make a call to someone who has supported you.

- *Say thank you* more often.

- *Have an ageless attitude.* Let it shine through your attitude and outlook.

Afterword

Congratulations on your new ageless journey! But I want to share a few thoughts before I leave you. Breakthroughs and discoveries in anti-aging medicine are happening at an unprecedented and exponential rate. The therapeutic arsenal to fight diseases is also rapidly expanding.

Sadly, that's not where things are in the twenty-first century. Hospitals and clinicians have yet to keep up with the speed of those discoveries. At present, they are buried in tons of paperwork, continuous computer upgrades, and insurance and government bureaucracies. In the United States, doctors spend 40 percent of their time filling out electronic records versus taking care of patients! They have to fill in tons of click data to finish notes that were done by hand in the past and approve patients for almost every medication and test. This is the allopathic medicine approach in a world of sickness and drugs. Health care in the United States is one big mess.

Many elderly people are filling hospitals and nursing homes with age-related diseases. Sadly, many of the elderly are just existing, not living. The costs of this bureaucracy and taking care of age-related diseases are astronomical.

My Vision of the Future of Aging

I have a few more dreams. We need a new direction to age differently. We need to change government guidelines on what is considered healthy.

Government guidelines should not include any fake foods. We need to educate doctors on pro-aging nutrition, anti-aging medications, and bioidentical hormones. There should be algorithms to follow to target all ten hallmarks of aging.

We also need futuristic gyms with exercise with oxygen therapy, cold plunges, cryotherapy, Power Plates, and infrared saunas.

We need insurance companies to consider *aging* a *disease*. The cost of the supplements and medications that slow aging should be covered by insurance companies. Pharmaceutical companies need to find molecules, medications, and peptides that can fight aging on the cellular level directly versus targeting age-related diseases. We need the FDA not to attack peptides, stem cells, and exosomes. People should not travel abroad to get those treatments. It is their choice. We need a revolution in health care—and maybe this book is the first step in that direction.

I thank you for picking up this book and reading through to the end. I am honored that you took the time to read what I have to say. I hope by now you have recognized how much power you have to enhance your health, endurance, appearance, and extend your life. It is your health, and it does not belong to anybody else. Your body, mind, and life force (spirit) work together. So does every cell of your body, communicating and working with your organs, bones, blood, and every solid and fluid that makes you—*you*.

You only have one life, so make the absolute best of it. Do not wait for anyone to lead you in the right direction; you are the one in charge. The future is already here. You now have the knowledge. You understand the biological explanations of how your body works, right down to the cellular and molecular level. It's time to put all this knowledge into action.

Forget all the mistakes of the past. Look to the future. As you progress toward radiant health and robust longevity, you'll see your body respond to your care.

Many people, when asked about their age, shave off a few years. No one wants to admit how old they really are. Yes, aging sucks. But I hope you realize that what matters is your biological age, and not your chronological age. I hope that I have helped you get younger as you followed some of my recommendations or all of them.

It has been my honor that you have allowed me to provide you with new knowledge, motivation, and inspiration. I truly thank you again for reading *The Ageless Revolution*. Remember to focus on the benefits of change and keep your eyes on the goal! Embrace the ageless challenge and, most of all, embrace life. Have a purpose, be happy, and live your best life now.

As I conclude *The Ageless Revolution*, let us share a toast, maybe with a glass of red wine: "To great health, staying younger longer, much longer, hopefully becoming a healthy centenarian, and truly living an ageless life."

Appendix

The Ageless Revolution Food Choices

Vegetables to Enjoy • 5–7 servings a day

Artichokes
Arugula
Asparagus
Bamboo shoots
Bell peppers (orange, green, red, yellow)
Broccoli
Brussels sprouts
Cabbage
Carrots
Celery
Chard

Cucumbers
Eggplant
Endive (chicory)
Greens (chard, collard, mustard, turnip)
Hot peppers
Kale
Leeks
Lettuce (all varieties)
Okra
Onions
Parsley

Radicchio
Radishes
Rutabaga
Scallions
Spinach
Sprouts (all varieties)
String beans
Sweet potatoes
Sweet purple potatoes
Turnips
Zucchini

Vegetables to Limit

Beets (avoid if you need to lose weight)

Potatoes (too starchy)

Fruits to Enjoy

Eat two fruits a day maximum. Note that some fruits are considered two servings. These include tropical fruits like mangoes, pineapples, and bananas, because they have an excess of fructose.

Acai berries	Cherries	Pears
Apple (two servings)	Cranberries	Pineapple (two
Banana (two servings)	Honeydew melon	servings)
Blackberries	Kiwi	Strawberries
Blueberries	Mango (two servings)	Tomatoes
Cantaloupe	Oranges	

Fruits to Avoid

Dried fruits   All fruit juices (except tomato juice)

Grains to Enjoy

Barley	Oatmeal (non-instant)	Whole-grain cereals
Bread (pumpernickel,	Rice (brown in small	with no added
rye, whole grain)	amounts, black,	sugar or chemicals
Corn (small amounts)	or wild with more	Whole wheat pasta
	fiber)	

Grains to Avoid

All refined grains	All pastries made with	All low-fat and fat-free
(white bread, white	white flour	products with
rice, white pasta)		added sugar,
		high-fructose corn
		syrup, and other
		chemicals

Protein

Go for more plant-based protein on *The Ageless Revolution*, such as beans and mushrooms. Also enjoy more seafood.

Protein to Enjoy

All shellfish	Legumes	Poultry (chicken,
Fish (halibut, herring,	Liver	Cornish game hen,
tuna, sardines, wild	Mushrooms	duck, turkey, goose,
salmon)		pheasant—organic)

Protein to Eat Sparingly • Once every two to three weeks:

Buffalo/bison burgers	Organic red meat, pork, and lamb are okay, but eat moderately or sparingly, since frequent consumption is linked to cancer when charcoal grilled. Have red meat as stew instead.	Limit tofu and tempeh as excess soy is linked to underactive thyroid. Two times a week is okay.

Protein to Avoid

Canned tuna in soybean oil (contains trans fats)	Nitrite-containing products like ham, hot dogs, bacon, bologna, Canadian bacon, and sausage. It's best to cut them out completely because of their strong link to many cancers. If you eat processed meats, go for the sea-salt-preserved variety.	Soy protein isolate, which is chemically treated with nitrites, is present in soy burgers, low-carb shakes, low-carb chocolate bars, and low-carb chocolates.
Cow brain (for the risk of mad cow disease)		

Dairy to Enjoy (Organic)

A small serving of full-fat milk or small piece of cheese

A splash of cream or organic whole milk (cow or goat) in decaffeinated beverages is acceptable, but limit dairy to one serving a day.
Cheddar cheese
Cottage cheese

Farmer's cheese
Feta cheese
Goat cheese
Kefir
Mozzarella cheese
Parmesan cheese
Ricotta cheese
Swiss cheese
Yogurt

Dairy to Avoid

American cheese (it's made with soybean oil)

Milk Substitutes to Enjoy (all unsweetened)

Almond milk

Cashew milk
Coconut milk

Oat milk

Milk Substitutes to Avoid

Rice milk (it contains excess sugar)

Soy milk (contains an excess of polyunsaturated oils)

Fat-free, 1%, 2% milk (void of fats that help you absorb the fat-soluble vitamins)

Nuts to Enjoy • **Eat a handful two to three times a week:**

Eat these nuts raw, no oils, not roasted or salted.
Nut butters are good if they are extracted organically, without the use of chemicals.

Almonds
Brazil nuts
Cashews (although they are technically fruit)
Hazelnuts

Macadamias
Pecans
Walnuts

Oils to Enjoy

Almond oil used cold on salads

Avocado oil for cooking and cold on salads

Extra-virgin olive oil can be used for light cooking and salads, but don't heat to elevated temperatures. Macadamia oil is useful in cooking.

Safflower and sunflower oils—unrefined, cold-pressed, and poly unsaturated—in small amounts to dress salads. Do not heat.

Fats to Enjoy

Remember the types of fats on *The Ageless Revolution* are all natural. No fake fats!

Avocado
Butter (organic)
Coconut

Dark chocolate made with real cocoa butter and reduced sugar. It's better to eat natural sugar in very small amounts than to use any artificial sweeteners.

Ghee (clarified butter for cooking if you don't like the taste of butter)
Palm oil

Fats to Avoid

All refined vegetable oils (corn, safflower, sunflower, soybean, mixed-vegetable oil)

Animal fat from nonorganic sources because they are likely to have toxins, hormones, antibiotics, and pesticides.

Non hydrogenated or liquid margarine
Partially hydrogenated oils and fats, fast-food oils, and margarine brands like I Can't Believe It's Not Butter!

Vegetable shortening

Good Sweeteners

Don't consume fake sweeteners on *The Ageless Revolution*. Artificial sweeteners are not natural to our bodies. I like stevia and monk fruit. Occasionally you can have manuka honey, in lesser amounts. If you use agave, it should be from the plant itself, not refined. Remember, excess fructose has a worse effect on our bodies than sugar. *Allulose* is a new sweetener that seems to be okay for now.

Sweeteners to Avoid

High-fructose corn syrup	Maple syrup	Refined agave
	Molasses	Sugar (white, brown)
	Regular honey	

Beverages to Enjoy

You can have several cups of tea a day, but limit coffee to one cup. Tea and herbal teas have an edge over coffee. Tea comes in a variety of types so have plenty in your kitchen cupboard. Enjoy black tea, green tea, chamomile tea, and jasmine tea with no added sugar. I love green tea, which has *epigallocatechin* (EGCG), one of the strongest antioxidants. Experiment with the different teas discussed in *The Ageless Revolution*.

What About Soda?

Stay away from all sodas and soft drinks. Research shows that drinking more than one regular or diet soda a day is associated with a cluster of risk factors linked to diabetes and heart disease. Soda also leaches calcium out of the bones, so it's linked to osteoporosis.

What About Alcohol?

Alcohol, in excess, is bad for your longevity. If you want to drink, alcohol should be consumed in moderation. Of course, the best alcoholic drink for longevity may be red wine because it has high levels of flavonoids.

Beverages to Enjoy

All vegetable juices except beet	Decaffeinated tea and coffee	Organic hot chocolate with no added sugar, in small amounts
Black tea	Lemonade sweetened with stevia	
Caffeinated herbal and green tea	Mineral water	Sparkling water
		Tomato juice

Beverages to Limit

Alcohol	Beet juice because it has excessive sugar	Coffee

Beverages to Avoid

All carbonated beverages including regular and diet soda	All fruit juices except tomato Energy drinks	Hot chocolate with added sugars and hydrogenated oils

Condiments, Spices, and Herbs to Enjoy

Black pepper	Dill	Paprika
Cajun blended seasonings	Fennel	Rosemary
	Garlic (best fresh)	Sea salt
Cardamom	Lemon	Tarragon
Cayenne pepper	Lime	Thyme
Ceylon cinnamon	Mayonnaise (made with olive oil)	Turmeric
Crushed red pepper flakes		Vanilla
	Nutmeg	Worcestershire sauce
Cumin	Onion	Za'atar
Curry powder	Oregano	

Spices to Limit

Regular salt

Condiments to Avoid

All fat-free salad dressings with added sugar, partially hydrogenated oils, or soybean oil Barbecue sauce with high-fructose corn syrup	Jellies or jams sweetened with high-fructose corn syrup Ketchup with high-fructose corn syrup	Mayonnaise made with soybean oil because it may have traces of trans fats

The Ageless Revolution
Diet Planner

Typical Day on *The Ageless Revolution*

BREAKFAST: 2-egg omelet, 1 slice of whole wheat toast with butter, 1 small cup of blueberries

LUNCH: a few grilled shrimp and a side salad, 1 tablespoon of olive oil

DINNER: grilled organic chicken thigh with mixed vegetables

BREAKFAST: full-fat organic Greek yogurt (no sugar) with live probiotics and a few strawberries

OPTIONAL MIDMORNING SNACK: turmeric almond latte

LUNCH: kale salad with salmon, toasted walnuts, and a few cranberries

DINNER: cauliflower cream soup, whole wheat croutons

BREAKFAST: 2 boiled organic eggs, 1 slice of cheese

LUNCH: ginger organic chicken, spinach salad with extra-virgin olive oil

OPTIONAL MIDAFTERNOON SNACK: ½ cup fruit with 2 teaspoons unsweetened whipped cream

DINNER: lentil soup, 2 whole wheat crackers

BREAKFAST: 1 cup mashed chickpeas on lettuce, a fruit cup

LUNCH: shrimp curry, 1 cup of wild rice

DINNER: salmon with 1 cup of steamed vegetables

BREAKFAST: 1 cup of organic non-instant oatmeal with ½ cup of almond milk

OPTIONAL MIDMORNING SNACK: 1 cup berries

LUNCH: nitrite-free turkey sandwich on whole wheat toast, small salad

DINNER: curried yellow lentils with fresh mint-cilantro sauce

---

BREAKFAST: 2-egg omelet with 2 nitrite-free turkey sausages, 2 slices whole wheat toast

OPTIONAL MIDMORNING SNACK: 1 or 2 small pieces of reduced-sugar dark chocolate

LUNCH: garlic chicken with 1 cup of steamed vegetables

OPTIONAL MIDAFTERNOON SNACK: ½ cup unsalted nuts

DINNER: 1 cup broccoli soup, grilled chicken breast.

BREAKFAST: organic omelet with vegetables

LUNCH: whole wheat pasta (4 scoops, the size of a tennis ball) with 1 cup of seafood

DINNER: veggie chili with 3 types of chiles, a side salad

BREAKFAST: egg frittata with 2 slices of sourdough bread, 1 teaspoon butter, 1 cup berries

OPTIONAL MIDMORNING SNACK: small matcha green latte with almond milk

LUNCH: saffron chicken with 1 cup wild rice

DINNER: 2 slices of vegetable, whole wheat, thin-crust pizza

BREAKFAST: acai bowl (acai berries, chia seeds), 2 boiled eggs

LUNCH: black beans with 1 cup of wild rice

DINNER: butternut squash curry soup with 2 whole wheat crackers, small salad

Intermittent Fasting Days Food Choices That Can Be Followed Between Regular Days

For Leangains and the 5:2 Fasting Plans

Sample Day 1

MORNING: 9 AM, iced water with electrolytes or tea with no milk

BRUNCH AT NOON: 2-egg organic omelet with 1 cup of blueberries

DINNER: 5 PM, grilled organic chicken thigh with 1 cup of mixed
  vegetables

Sample Day 2

MORNING: 9 AM, iced water with electrolytes

BRUNCH AT NOON: a full-fat organic yogurt with 1 cup of berries

DINNER: 5 PM, grilled salmon, side salad tossed with walnuts,
  and 1 teaspoon of olive oil

Sample Day 3

BREAKFAST AT NOON: a keto coffee (coffee made with butter)

DINNER: 6 PM, shrimp and bean mixed salad and 1 cup fruit for dessert

---

Sample Day 4

MORNING: 10 AM, a large unsweetened black iced tea

DINNER: 6 PM, grilled salmon with 2 cups of mixed vegetables

Add-On Treatments for Various Medical Conditions

Alzheimer's Disease

Ashwagandha 125 mg daily

Sage blueberry 200 mg a day

Squid oil with DHA and EPA

Nattokinase 100 mg a day

N-acetylcysteine (NAC) 2.5 grams a day

L-serine 12 grams a day

Nicotinamide riboside 1 gram a day

L-carnitine 3 grams a day

Intermittent fasting

A peptide called cerebrolysin

Arthritis

Niacinamide 3 grams a day divided into 3 doses

Borage oil

Exosomes intravenously

Attention Deficit Hyperactivity Disorder (ADHD)

Exosomes intravenously

Peptide called selank

Decreased Sexual Desire in Women

A peptide called *bremelanotide* sold in pharmacies as a drug called Vyleesi, 1.75 mg subcutaneous 45 minutes before sex

Depression

5-hydroxytryptophan

Saffron pill (works better than antidepressants and without weight gain)

Diabetes

Dihydroberberine 150 mg orally twice a day

Hesperidin 500 mg daily

Gynostemma extract 450 mg daily

Elevated Cholesterol

Red yeast extract

Nattokinase 100–300 mg daily

Heart Disease

Take vitamin K2, 45 mcg orally daily

Enhanced external counterpulsation (EECP)

Nattokinase 100–300 mg a day
Red yeast extract

Joint Pain

A peptide called BPC 157

Hypertension

An amino acid called taurine 500–3,000 mg a day

Ischemic Stroke

Hyperbaric oxygen chamber

Enhanced external counterpulsation (EECP)

A peptide called cerebrolysin

Obesity

Follow a balanced diet

Eliminate sugar

GLP-1 peptides injection with medical supervision

Osteoporosis

Calcium citrate 500 mg three times a day

Vitamin K2 45 mcg a day

Weight-bearing exercise

Parkinson's Disease

| Glutathione drip (an infusion) | Hyperbaric oxygen chamber | NAD exosomes |

Urinary Tract Infection

D-mannose 1.5 grams twice a day for 3 days, then once daily for 10 days

---

To get many of the supplements in *The Ageless Revolution*,
call **Life Extension** at **1-888-543-5441** and give them
code **Ageless Rx** for discounts.

The Ageless Revolution
Recipes

Berry Yogurt Parfait with Chocolate Nuts

SERVES 2 (with about 4 cups of leftover chocolate nuts)

The chocolate nuts also make for a flavorful, satisfying, and convenient snack.

¼ cup plus 2 teaspoons monk fruit sweetener, divided

¼ cup extra-virgin olive oil

1 large egg

3 tablespoons unsweetened cocoa powder

1½ teaspoons vanilla extract, divided

1 teaspoon kosher salt

½ teaspoon ground cinnamon

2 cups unsalted raw walnuts

1 ¾ cups unsalted raw pecans

1 cup unsweetened/plain Greek full-fat yogurt

1 cup mixture of fresh raspberries and blueberries

1. Preheat the oven to 325°F and line a large baking sheet with parchment paper. In a large bowl, whisk together ¼ cup of the monk fruit sweetener, oil, egg, cocoa, 1 teaspoon of the vanilla, and the salt and cinnamon. Add nuts and, using tongs, coat thoroughly in the chocolate mixture. Pour onto the

baking sheet and bake until aromatic, crisp, and darker in color, for about 18 minutes. Let cool.

2. In a small bowl, mix yogurt with the remaining 2 teaspoons monk fruit sweetener and ½ teaspoon vanilla. Spoon into two parfait glasses or bowls. Top each portion with berries. Sprinkle ¼ cup of the chocolate nuts on top of each portion.

Greek Eggs Scramble with Tomatoes and Feta

SERVES 2

Feel free to use other vegetables, such as diced bell peppers or sliced mushrooms. Just be sure to sauté them first.

1 teaspoon extra-virgin olive oil, divided	6 large eggs
1 large clove garlic, minced (about 1 heaping teaspoon)	Black pepper to taste
5-ounce bag fresh baby spinach	1 Roma tomato, halved, seeded, and chopped (about ½ cup)
¼ teaspoon kosher salt, divided	¼ cup crumbled feta cheese

1. In a medium nonstick sauté pan, pour half the oil and heat over medium. Add garlic and sauté just until aromatic, for 1–2 minutes. Add spinach plus ⅛ teaspoon of the salt and sauté until fully wilted, turning with tongs, for about 2 minutes. Use tongs to transfer spinach to a paper towel–lined plate to drain.

2. In a medium bowl, whisk eggs with the remaining ⅛ teaspoon salt plus the pepper. Pour the remaining ½ teaspoon oil in the same pan and heat over medium-low. When warm, add the egg mix and cook, stirring frequently with a wooden spoon, until almost cooked through, for about 4 minutes. Use tongs to stir in the cooked spinach, tomato, and feta. Serve immediately.

Frittata Muffins

MAKES 12 (4–6 servings)

Prepare one batch, and you'll have breakfast for four days. Be sure to use a non-stick muffin pan for easy cleanup. For the most colorful frittata muffins, include red and orange bell peppers.

Olive oil cooking spray
1 teaspoon avocado or olive oil
2 teaspoons minced garlic
  (about 1 large clove)
1–1½ teaspoons minced jalapeño
2 bell peppers, diced (about 2 cups)
5 ounces white button mushrooms, stems removed, and caps thinly sliced (about 2 cups)

1 teaspoon salt, divided
14 grinds black pepper, divided
12 large eggs
1 cup shredded cheddar cheese
  (about 3 ounces)
½ cup finely chopped, fresh, flat-leaf parsley leaves

1. Preheat the oven to 350°F and spray a standard 12-cup muffin pan (nonstick or silicone) with cooking spray. Heat oil in a large nonstick sauté pan over medium heat. When warm, add the garlic and jalapeño and sauté until aromatic, for about 2 minutes (don't let garlic brown). Add peppers, mushrooms, ½ teaspoon of salt, and 8 grinds of the pepper, and sauté until the peppers soften, for 8–10 minutes. Pour the sautéed vegetables onto a paper towel–lined plate to drain.

2. In a large bowl, whisk together the remaining ½ teaspoon salt and 6 grinds of pepper plus eggs, cheddar, and parsley. Add the cooked vegetables and mix well. Ladle the egg mixture evenly into the muffin cups.

3. Bake until the eggs are just set (their centers should spring back when touched) and the frittata muffins are lightly golden brown, for 15–20 minutes. Let cool for about 15 minutes before cutting around their edges to release them from the pan.

Keto Coffee

SERVES 1

2 cups coffee

2 tablespoons grass-fed butter or coconut oil

1 tablespoon sugar-free, heavy whipping cream (optional)

1 teaspoon vanilla extract (optional)

1. Brew coffee using your favorite beans or coffee grounds.
2. Pour coffee into a blender or your mug.
3. Add 2 tablespoons of butter.
4. Add whipping cream and vanilla extract if using.
5. Blend or use a handheld frothing device to mix until a frothy head forms.

Lunch and Dinner

Cauliflower Cream Soup

SERVES 3–4

1 large head cauliflower (about 2 pounds cut in small florets)

2 tablespoons extra-virgin olive oil

1 medium red onion

5 cloves garlic, peeled and minced

4 cups chicken broth (32 ounces)

2 tablespoons butter

2 sprigs fresh thyme

3 cups milk

Pinch sea salt

¼ teaspoon black pepper

1 tablespoon fresh lemon juice

1. Chop cauliflower florets into small pieces.
2. Heat olive oil in a large stock pot over medium heat, add the onion and sauté for 5 minutes until it is soft and translucent. Stir in garlic and sauté for 2 more minutes.
3. Add chopped cauliflower, chicken broth, butter, and thyme, and stir to combine. Continue to cook until the mixture reaches a simmer.
4. Lower the heat and continue simmering for another 20–25 minutes or until the cauliflower is tender.
5. Transfer mixture to the blender. Purée the soup until it is smooth.
6. Add milk to the mixture in the blender.
7. Serve immediately; season to taste with salt, pepper, and lemon.

Cream of Mushroom Soup

SERVES 5–6

5 cups sliced fresh mushrooms

1½ cups chicken broth

½ cup chopped onion

⅛ teaspoon dried thyme

3 tablespoons butter

3 tablespoons whole wheat flour

¼ teaspoon sea salt

¼ teaspoon ground black pepper

1 cup half-and-half

1. Simmer mushrooms, broth, onion, and thyme in a large heavy saucepan until vegetables are tender, for 10–15 minutes.
2. Carefully transfer the hot mixture to a blender or food processor. Cover and hold lid. Blend until nearly smooth.
3. Melt butter in the same saucepan. Whisk in flour until smooth. Whisk in salt and pepper. Slowly whisk in half-and-half, and then the mushroom mixture.
4. Bring soup to a boil and cook, stirring constantly, until thickened.
5. Taste and season with more sea salt and pepper if needed.

Saffron Chicken

SERVES 4

8 pieces chicken thighs and drumsticks

Salt and pepper to season

2 tablespoons grapeseed oil

2 tablespoons butter

1 large onion, peeled and chopped

3 cloves garlic minced

2 teaspoon minced ginger

½ teaspoon paprika

¼ teaspoon ground cayenne pepper

1 large chicken bouillon cube, crushed

2 tablespoons whole wheat flour

2 cups chicken broth

¼ teaspoon saffron threads

3 tablespoons parsley plus extra for garnishing

1. Sprinkle chicken with salt and pepper.
2. Heat a pan on medium-high heat and put the grapeseed oil in the pan.
3. Add chicken pieces to the pan when oil is heated. Let chicken pieces brown on one side, then turn pieces to brown on the other sides.
4. Remove chicken when browned and set aside.
5. Add butter to the pan, then add onion. Let onion cook until translucent.
6. Stir in garlic and ginger followed by paprika, cayenne, and crushed soup cube. Stir until fragrant.
7. Add whole wheat flour and mix until fully incorporated, then pour in chicken broth and mix.
8. Stir in saffron threads. Add parsley, then turn heat down to low.
9. Return chicken to the pan, place a lid on it, and let simmer for 35 to 45 minutes or until chicken is tender.
10. Top with additional parsley. Serve with salad or mixed vegetables.

Salmon with Za'atar
and Sweet Purple Potatoes

SERVES 4–5

12 small sweet purple potatoes
(about 12 ounces), scrubbed

2 cups grape tomatoes (about 10
ounces), halved if you like

6 ounces broccoli florets

2 tablespoons extra-virgin olive oil

Pinch of sea salt

Pinch of pepper

3 tablespoons fresh minced garlic
(5 to 6 cloves), divided

2 teaspoons za'atar spice, divided

1 teaspoon ground coriander, divided

1 pound wild salmon filet, no skin

1 lemon, cut into quarters

1. Preheat the oven to 400°F.
2. In a large bowl, place the sweet purple potatoes, grape tomatoes, and broccoli. Pour in extra-virgin olive oil. Add salt, pepper, 1 tablespoon minced garlic, 1 teaspoon za'atar spice, and ½ teaspoon coriander. Toss again so that the spices are distributed evenly to coat the vegetables. Transfer the vegetables to a large baking sheet with a rim.
3. Pat salmon dry. Season with salt and pepper. Drizzle on just a little extra-virgin olive oil. Spread remaining garlic evenly on top. Sprinkle on remaining za'atar and coriander.
4. Cut seasoned salmon into 4 equal pieces, and place on the prepared baking sheet with the vegetables. Add another drizzle of extra-virgin olive oil over the salmon and veggies.
5. Bake in a heated oven for 15 minutes. Remove from heat and squeeze lemon juice on salmon. Sprinkle more za'atar all over. Enjoy with your favorite salad or some wild rice.

Miso-and-Lime-Glazed Salmon with Black Pepper

SERVES 2

This delicious entrée is special enough for company but comes together in mere minutes.

1 tablespoon fresh lime juice	2 teaspoons monk fruit sweetener
1 tablespoon miso paste, such as mellow white	2 (6-ounce) salmon filets, pin bones removed
1 tablespoon low-sodium soy sauce	Black pepper to taste

1. Preheat the oven to 400°F. Line a small baking sheet with parchment paper. In a small bowl, whisk together lime, miso, soy, and monk fruit until smooth.
2. Place salmon filets skin side down on the baking sheet. Spoon the glaze evenly on top, then sprinkle each filet with 4 grinds of pepper. Roast until just opaque, for about 12 minutes.

Chicken Curry with Cardamom

SERVES 6–8

5 tablespoons grapeseed oil

2 pieces (2-inch) cinnamon sticks

8 cardamom pods

3 pounds of chicken, cut into 12 pieces

1 small onion, chopped

2 cloves garlic, peeled and chopped

2 tablespoons coriander

1 tablespoon curcumin

½ teaspoon turmeric

½ teaspoon cayenne pepper

2 medium tomatoes, chopped

4 cups chicken stock

Pinch of sea salt (optional)

1. Put the oil in a large, wide sauté pan over high heat. When hot, put in the cinnamon and cardamom. A few seconds later, put in some of the chicken pieces and brown them until golden on all sides. Transfer to a bowl, leaving the whole spices in the pan. Brown the remaining chicken in the same way and add to the bowl.
2. Add the onions to the pan, lower the heat to medium, and sauté until they start to brown lightly at the edges. Add the garlic and stir a few times.
3. Now add the coriander, curcumin, turmeric, and cayenne pepper. Stir once or twice.
4. Put in the tomatoes, stirring until they begin to soften.
5. Return the browned chicken and all its accumulated juices to the pan, along with the chicken stock, add a pinch of salt if the stock is not salted, and bring to a boil. Cover and cook somewhat rapidly over medium heat for 15 minutes.
6. Remove the cover and turn the heat to high. Cook, stirring now and then, until the sauce has thickened.

Roasted Chicken Thighs
with Lemon-Garlic-Herb Butter

SERVES 2–3 (Makes 6 thighs)

Ideal for holiday meals, this entree derives its deliciousness from a quick home-made lemon-garlic-herb butter. For ease, zest the lemon, then halve and juice.

2 tablespoons unsalted butter, at room temperature

1 tablespoon plus 2 teaspoons finely chopped fresh sage leaves (about 12 leaves)

1 tablespoon minced garlic (about 2 large cloves)

2 teaspoons finely chopped fresh rosemary

1 teaspoon freshly grated lemon zest (from one lemon)

1 teaspoon salt, divided

Black pepper (24 grinds divided)

6 boneless, skinless chicken thighs

1 tablespoon fresh lemon juice

1. Preheat the oven to 400°F and line a large baking sheet with parchment paper. In a small bowl, use your hands to massage together butter, sage, garlic, rosemary, zest, ½ tsp of salt, and 12 grinds of pepper.
2. Place chicken thighs on the baking sheet and rub both sides evenly with the butter. Then sprinkle both sides evenly with the remaining ½ teaspoon salt and 12 grinds of pepper.
3. Roast until opaque and slightly golden, for about 35 minutes. Transfer chicken to a large bowl. Carefully pour and scrape the meat juices and herb butter solids into the bowl. Add the lemon juice and, using tongs, gently toss. Serve immediately.

Chicken Cauliflower Fried Rice

SERVES 2

This easy weeknight dinner is flavorful and reminiscent of your favorite Chinese takeout. For even more convenience, you can pour the riced cauliflower in the pan straight from the freezer. The carrots add color and sweetness; however, if you are watching your sugar, feel free to omit them.

¼ cup plus 1 tablespoon low-sodium soy sauce

1 teaspoon monk fruit sweetener

1 tablespoon avocado oil, divided

1 pound boneless skinless chicken breasts, cut into 1-inch pieces

½ cup thinly sliced green onion (about 3)

½ cup peeled and finely chopped carrot (about 1)

2 teaspoons minced garlic

2 teaspoons peeled and minced ginger

10-ounce bag frozen cauliflower rice

1. In a medium bowl, whisk together the soy sauce and monk fruit.
2. Heat 2 teaspoons of oil in a medium sauté pan over medium-high heat. When hot, add the chicken and sauté until golden and cooked through, for about 8 minutes. Transfer chicken and juices to a bowl.
3. To the hot pan, pour the remaining teaspoon of oil and the onion, carrot, garlic, and ginger, and sauté, scraping the bottom of the pan to release any brown bits, for about 2 minutes (do not let burn). Pour in the soy sauce mixture and bring to a boil over high heat, continuing to scrape the bottom of the pan.
4. Stir in the chicken, chicken juices, and cauliflower rice and sauté, breaking up the cauliflower rice and stirring the dish, until the carrots are tender and the dish is hot, in about 5 minutes.

Veggie Chili with Three Types of Chiles

Serves 6–8

For a more flavorful, thick chili, prepare a day ahead. Serve topped with yogurt mixed with freshly grated lime zest and chopped avocado.

1 tablespoon avocado oil

2 cups chopped red and yellow bell peppers (about 2)

2 cups chopped red onion (about 1)

1 tablespoon chopped garlic (about 3 cloves)

2 teaspoons chopped jalapeño

2½ kosher salt, divided

2 teaspoons ground cumin, divided

2 teaspoons ground chipotle or ancho chili powder (not a blend), divided

½ teaspoon cinnamon, divided

Black pepper to taste

1 quart low-sodium vegetable broth

28-ounce can whole plum tomatoes

2 (15.5-ounce) cans pinto beans, drained and rinsed

15.5-ounce can black beans, drained and rinsed

1 pound bag frozen peas

4-ounce can green chiles

1 tablespoon plus 2 teaspoons monk fruit sweetener

1. Heat oil in a Dutch oven over medium heat. When warm, add the bell peppers, onion, garlic, jalapeño, and half of the salt, cumin, chili powder, cinnamon, and black pepper. Cover and cook until softened, in about 4 minutes.

2. Stir in the broth, tomatoes, pinto beans, black beans, peas, green chiles, monk fruit, and remaining salt, cumin, chili powder, cinnamon, and black pepper. Bring to a boil over high heat, then cover and simmer over medium-low heat for 30 minutes.

Classic Beef Stew with Rosemary and Garlic

SERVES 4

This stew is even more delicious prepared a day or two ahead. Serve over mashed cauliflower for a homey meal. To reduce the sugar, feel free to double the onions and omit the carrots.

2 pounds beef chuck stew meat, in 2-inch pieces

2 tablespoons whole wheat flour

1¼ teaspoons kosher salt, divided

Black pepper to taste

1 tablespoon plus 1 teaspoon avocado oil, divided

1 cup chopped red onion (about ½ large)

1 cup peeled and chopped carrot (about 2)

1 tablespoon finely chopped garlic plus 1 peeled large garlic clove, divided

¾ cup fruity red wine, such as Merlot or Zinfandel

2 tablespoons tomato paste

1 teaspoon Dijon mustard

1 cup low-sodium chicken or beef stock

4 sprigs fresh rosemary, tied together with kitchen twine

½ tablespoon unsalted butter

8 ounces white button mushrooms, stems trimmed, and caps quartered (2 cups)

1. Preheat the oven to 350°F. In a large bowl, toss beef with flour, 1 teaspoon of salt, and the pepper. Heat 2 teaspoons of the oil in a Dutch oven over medium-high heat. When hot, pour in all the beef and seasoned flour and sauté, turning with tongs, until brown on all sides, in 8 or 9 minutes. Transfer the meat and juice to a plate.

2. Add remaining 2 teaspoons of oil to the Dutch oven. Add the onion, carrot, and 1 tablespoon chopped garlic and sauté for 2 minutes, scraping brown bits off the bottom of the pan (do not let them burn).

3. Add the wine, tomato paste, and mustard, and bring to a boil over high heat, continuing to scrape the pan bottom. Stir in the stock and rosemary. Return the meat and meat juices to the pot, submerging the meat in the sauce. Cover the pot. Carefully transfer to the oven and cook until the meat is fork-tender, in 1¾–2 hours. Fish out and discard the rosemary.

4. About 15 minutes before the meat is ready, melt the butter over medium heat in a medium sauté pan. Add the mushrooms, remaining ¼ teaspoon salt, and whole garlic clove and sauté until the mushrooms turn golden brown, soften, and release their juices, in 6–7 minutes. Discard the garlic. Stir the mushrooms into the stew and serve immediately.

Curried Yellow Lentils
with Fresh Mint-Cilantro Sauce

MAKES ABOUT 6 CUPS LENTILS plus 1 cup sauce

*This satisfying, flavorful main dish should last you for three lunches or dinners.
If you do not like cilantro, feel free to use fresh, flat-leaf parsley instead.*

LENTILS:

- 2 teaspoons avocado oil
- 1 cup chopped red onion
- 1 tablespoon thinly sliced garlic (about 2 large cloves)
- 1 tablespoon peeled and finely chopped fresh ginger root
- 2 teaspoons yellow curry powder
- ¼ teaspoon ground turmeric
- Black pepper to taste
- 4.5-oz tube tomato paste
- 2 tablespoons unsweetened tamarind paste or concentrate
- 2 cups dried yellow lentils
- 1 quart low-sodium vegetable stock
- 2 teaspoons monk fruit sweetener
- 1 teaspoon kosher salt

SAUCE:

- ½ cup fresh cilantro leaves
- ¼ cup fresh mint leaves
- 1½ teaspoons monk fruit sweetener
- ½ teaspoon fresh lemon juice
- ¼ teaspoon kosher salt

1. FOR THE LENTILS: Heat oil in a medium saucepan over medium heat. When warm, add the onion, garlic, ginger, curry powder, turmeric, and pepper, and sauté until the onion softens, in about 4 minutes (do not let burn). Stir in the tomato paste and tamarind and sauté for another minute. Stir in the lentils, stock, monk fruit sweetener, and salt, and bring to a boil over high heat. Cover and simmer over medium-low heat until the lentils are cooked through, in about 30 minutes. Stir in 1 cup warm water to thin.

2. FOR THE SAUCE: In a high-speed blender or food processor, place all ingredients plus 1 cup water and puree until smooth, for about 1 minute. Drizzle sauce over the lentils when serving.

Berry Salad with Toasted Almonds, Goat Cheese, and Basil

SERVES 2

For the most flavorful and crisp greens, wash and spin the lettuce in advance. Then store in a plastic bag with a paper towel in the fridge for at least an hour.

¼ cup minced red onion

2 tablespoons fresh lemon juice

2 tablespoons extra-virgin olive oil

2 teaspoons monk fruit sweetener

¼ teaspoon salt, divided

Black pepper to taste (8 grinds, divided)

1 small head green leaf lettuce, cored and leaves torn into bite-size pieces (about 4 cups), washed, and spun dry

8 large fresh basil leaves, thinly sliced (about 3 tablespoons)

2 tablespoons blanched slivered almonds, lightly toasted

2½ ounces crumbled fresh goat cheese

½ cup fresh raspberries

1. In a medium bowl, stir together the onion and juice and let sit for 10 minutes. Then whisk in the oil, monk fruit sweetener, ⅛ teaspoon of the salt, and 4 grinds of the pepper.
2. In a large bowl, place the lettuce, basil, remaining salt, and remaining pepper, and toss until the greens are coated. Divide the greens between two plates.
3. Onto each plate, sprinkle half of the almonds, cheese, and raspberries. Serve immediately.

Kale Salad with Parmesan, Toasted Walnuts, and Grapes

SERVES 2 (Makes 5 tablespoons dressing)

Ideally, prepare this salad half an hour in advance so the kale has a chance to wilt. If you can find bagged shredded kale, feel free to use it instead. If not, be sure to remove any stems and to tear or slice leaves into bite-size pieces. For convenience, look for pre-grated Parmigiano-Reggiano cheese.

2 tablespoons minced red onion

2 tablespoons fresh lemon juice

2 tablespoons extra-virgin olive oil

1¼ teaspoons monk fruit sweetener

1 teaspoon Dijon mustard

½ teaspoon kosher salt, divided

Black pepper to taste (12 grinds, divided)

6 cups shredded or torn fresh kale leaves

½ cup red grapes (about 12), halved

9 baby tomatoes (green), halved

¼ cup finely grated Parmigiano-Reggiano cheese

¼ cup raw unsalted walnuts, lightly toasted and chopped

1. In a medium jar, place the onion, juice, oil, monk fruit, mustard, ¼ teaspoon salt, and 4 grinds of pepper. Cover and shake until creamy.
2. In a large bowl, use tongs to toss together the remaining ¼ teaspoon salt, 8 grinds of pepper, kale, grapes, tomatoes, and cheese. Divide between two plates and top each portion with nuts.

Sweets, Snacks, and Shakes

Spiced Nuts with Butter and Rosemary

MAKES 1–1½ CUPS

These easy-to-prepare nuts make for a decadent snack or sweet treat.

2 tablespoons unsalted butter, melted

2 tablespoons monk fruit sweetener

1 teaspoon finely chopped fresh
   rosemary

1 teaspoon kosher salt

¼ teaspoon ground cinnamon

⅛ teaspoon ground cayenne

Black pepper to taste

½ cup each raw, unsalted pistachios,
   walnuts, and pecans

1. Preheat the oven to 300°F and line a baking sheet with parchment paper.
   In a medium bowl, whisk together melted butter, monk fruit, rosemary, salt,
   cinnamon, cayenne, and black pepper. Add the nuts and toss well until
   coated.
2. Pour onto the baking sheet in one layer and roast until golden brown and
   aromatic, for about 15 minutes.

Ginger-Turmeric Latte

SERVES 2 (Makes about 2 cups)

This caffeine-free beverage is flavorful and crammed with healthful spices. Just know that, thanks to its yellow-orange color, it can stain.

2 cups unsweetened almond or other acceptable milk

1–2 tablespoons monk fruit sweetener to taste

1-inch piece fresh ginger root, peeled

½ teaspoon ground turmeric

¼ teaspoon ground Ceylon cinnamon

⅛ teaspoon kosher salt

1. Place all ingredients in a small heavy saucepan and bring to a boil over high heat, whisking occasionally. The second the mixture comes to a boil, turn off the heat (do not let the pot boil over). Remove and discard the ginger. Either froth with a handheld frother or carefully pour into a blender and blend until frothy, for about 10 seconds. Ladle into two mugs and serve immediately.

Whole-Grain Almond Chocolate Chip Cookies

MAKES ABOUT 19 COOKIES

These should remind you of your favorite soft chocolate chip cookies—but with the nuttiness and nourishment of whole wheat flour. For the best results, make sure the almond butter is at room temperature.

2 cups whole wheat flour

1 teaspoon kosher salt

½ teaspoon baking soda

½ teaspoon baking powder

2 sticks unsalted butter, cubed

¼ cup unsweetened unsalted almond butter, well-stirred

1 cup Lakanto Classic Sweetener or Lakanto Baking Sweetener

¼ cup plus 1 tablespoon Lakanto Brown Sweetener or Lakanto Golden Sweetener

2 large eggs

1 teaspoon almond extract

1 teaspoon vanilla extract

9-ounce bag stevia-sweetened dark chocolate chips

1. Preheat the oven to 350°F and place racks on the upper and lower thirds. Line two large baking sheets with parchment paper.
2. In a large bowl, sift together flour, salt, baking soda, and baking powder.
3. In the bowl of a standing mixer (or with a large bowl and handheld mixer), cream together butter, almond butter, and two sugars on medium-high speed. Beat until well mixed, occasionally scraping down the sides of the bowl, for about 2 minutes. Add the eggs and extracts and beat for another minute, scraping down the sides of the bowl again if necessary. Add the flour mixture and beat on medium-low just until incorporated, in about 10 seconds. Stir in chocolate chips by hand.
4. Using a ¼-cup measure, divide dough into balls and place on two baking sheets, spacing them 3 inches apart. Flatten each with your hand. Bake just until lightly golden brown on the edges, rotating baking sheet positions halfway through, for 13–16 minutes total (do not overbake). Let cool for 10 minutes.

Flourless Dark Chocolate Almond Cake with Raspberry Chia Preserves

SERVES 8. Makes a 9-inch-diameter cake and 1–1¼ cups preserves.

For the richest cake, I use a European-style butter (which has a higher fat content). Slather any remaining preserves on your morning whole-grain toast.

Nonstick cooking spray made with grapeseed oil

1½ cups superfine almond flour

¼ cup plus 2 tablespoons unsweetened cocoa powder

2 teaspoons baking powder

1¼ teaspoons kosher salt, divided

½ teaspoon ground cinnamon

½ cup plus ⅓ cup golden monk fruit sweetener, divided

3 large eggs

½ stick unsalted European-style butter, such as Kerrygold, melted

¼ cup unsweetened almond milk

1½ teaspoons pure vanilla extract

12-ounces fresh or 1 bag frozen raspberries

2 tablespoons chia seeds

1 tablespoon fresh lemon juice

1. Preheat the oven to 350°F and grease a 9-inch round cake pan with cooking spray. Line with a parchment paper circle and spray the parchment with more cooking spray.

2. In a large bowl, whisk together the almond flour, cocoa, baking powder, ¾ teaspoon of the salt, and cinnamon, removing as many lumps as possible.

3. In a medium bowl, whisk together ⅓ cup of the monk fruit, eggs, melted butter, milk, and vanilla until smooth. Add to the dry mix and stir with a wooden spoon just until combined.

4. Pour batter into the cake pan and spread with a spatula, banging the bottom of the pan against the counter a few times to distribute the batter evenly. Bake until a toothpick inserted in the center of the cake comes out clean, in about 16 minutes (check after 14 minutes).

5. Meanwhile, place the raspberries, remaining ½ cup monk fruit, chia seeds, lemon juice, and remaining ½ teaspoon salt in a medium saucepan and bring to a boil over high heat. Boil, stirring occasionally, until slightly thickened, in 3–4 minutes. Set it aside. Serve slices of cake with the preserves.

Snacks on the Run

Strawberry Vanilla Shake

MAKES 2 CUPS

For the most flavor, use the sweetest, highest-quality strawberries.

1 cup unsweetened vanilla almond milk

1 cup fresh or frozen strawberries (about 10)

½ cup unsweetened full-fat yogurt, such as almond or cow

2 tablespoons monk fruit sweetener or to taste

1. Place ingredients in a blender and blend until smooth, for about 1 minute.

Chocolate Almond Butter Shake

MAKES 1½ CUPS

For the ideal texture, drink the shake immediately. If the almond butter you use does not have salt, add ¼ teaspoon salt to the recipe.

1 cup unsweetened vanilla almond milk

¼ cup plus 2 tablespoons stevia-sweetened chocolate chips

¼ cup unsweetened salted almond butter

1 tablespoon whole flaxseeds

1. Place ingredients plus two ice cubes in a blender and blend until smooth, for about 2 minutes (make sure the chips purée).

Bibliography

Horvath, Steve. "Methylation Age of Human Tissues and Cell Types." *Genome Biology*, 14 (2013):3156.

Nesse, R.M. "Life Table Tests of Evolutionary Theories of Senescence." *Experimental Gerontology* (1988).

Carey, James R., Judge, Debra S. "Longevity Records: Life Spans of Mammals, Birds, Amphibians, Reptiles, and Fish." *Odense Monographs on Population Aging*, Denmark: Odense University Press, 2000.

"What Is Your Actual Age?" *Northwestern Medicine*, Chicago, June 2022. https://www.nm.org/healthbeat/medical-advances/science-and-research /What -is-Your-Actual-Age.

Furman, David, Campisi, Judith, Verdin, Eric, et al. "Chronic Inflammation in the Etiology of Disease Across the LifeSpan." *Nature Medicine*, December 2019. https://www.nature.com/articles/s41591-019-0675-0.

Hampton, Tracy. "Longevity Analysis Identifies 8 Key Social Factors." *Harvard Gazette*. February 2023. https://news.harvard.edu/gazette/story/2023/02 /how-long-will-you-live-8-social-factors-are-key/.

Buettner, Dan. *The Blue Zones: Lessons for Living Longer from the People Who've Lived the Longest.* National Geographic Books, Washington, DC, 2008.

McKay, D.L., Blumberg, J.B. "The Role of Tea in Human Health: An Update." *Journal of the American College of Nutrition*, 21(1), (2002):1–13.

Chacko, S.M., Thambi, P.T., Kuttan, R., Nishigaki, I. "Beneficial Effects of Green Tea: A Literature Review." *Chinese Medicine*, 5 (2010):13.

"Unprocessed Red and Processed Meats and Risk of Coronary Artery Disease and Type 2 Diabetes—an Updated Review of the Evidence." *Current Atherosclerosis Reports*, 14(6) (December 2012);14(6):515–24.

Caramia, G. "The Essential Fatty Acids Omega-6 and Omega-3: From Their Discovery to Their Use in Therapy." *Minerva Pediatrics*, 60(2) (2008):219–33.

Richopoulou, A., Costacou, T., Bamia, C., et al. "Adherence to a Mediterranean Diet and Survival in a Greek Population." *New England Journal of Medicine*, 2003 June 26;348(26):2599–608.

"Caloric Restriction: Implications for Human Cardiometabolic Health." *Journal of Cardiopulmonary Rehabilitation and Prevention*, 33(4) (July–August 2013):201-8.

Christensen, Kaare, Thinggaard, Mikael, McGue, Matt, et al. "Perceived Age as Clinically Useful Biomarker of Ageing: Cohort Study." *BMJ*, December 2009. https://pubmed.ncbi.nlm.nih.gov/20008378/.

Tzu-Wei, Lin, Sheng-Feng, Tsai, Yu-Min, Kuo. "Physical Exercise Enhances Neuroplasticity and Delays Alzheimer's Disease." *Brain Plasticity*, September 2018. https://www.ncbi.nlm.nih.gov/labs/pmc/articles/PMC6296269.

Memory and Aging Project, Rush University, Chicago. This is an ongoing study. https://www.rushu.rush.edu/research/departmental-research/memory-and -aging-project.

Irwin, Michael R., Vitiello, Michael V. "Implications of Sleep Disturbances and Inflammation for Alzheimer's Disease Dementia." *Lancet Neurology*, (March 2019). https://pubmed.ncbi.nlm.nih.gov/30661858/.

DePolo, Jamie. "Older Biological Age Compared to Chronological Age Linked to Increased Breast Cancer Risk." BreastCancer.org, February 2019. https://www.breastcancer.org/research-news/biological-vs-chronological -age -and-risk.

Jazwinski, Michal S., Sangkyu, Kim. "Examinations of the Dimensions of Biological Age." *Frontiers in Genetics*, (March 2019). https://www.frontiersin.org/articles/10.3389/fgene.2019.00263/full.

Wu, Julia W., Yakub, Amber, Yuan, Ma, et al. "Biological Age in Healthy Elderly Predicts Aging-Related Diseases Including Dementia." *Scientific Reports*, (August 2021). https://www.nature.com/articles/s41598-021-95425-5.

"What Is Epigenetics?" Centers for Disease Control and Prevention. https://www.cdc.gov/genomics/disease/epigenetics.htm.

Modig, K., Talback, M., Torssander, J., Ahlbom, A. "Payback Time? Influence of Having Children on Mortality in Old Age." *Journal of Epidemiology & Community Health* (2017). https://jech.bmj.com/content/71/5/424.

Salminen, A., Kaarniranta, K. "AMP-Activated Protein Kinase (AMPK) Controls the Aging Process via an Integrated Signaling Network." *Ageing Research Reviews*, 11(2) (April 2012):230–41.

Rojas, J., Arraiz, N., Aguirre, M., et al. "AMPK as Target for Intervention in Childhood and Adolescent Obesity." *Journal of Obesity* (2011):252817.

Chalkiadaki, A., Guarente, L. "High-Fat Diet Triggers Inflammation-Induced Cleavage of SIRT1 in Adipose Tissue to Promote Metabolic Dysfunction." *Cell Metabolism*, 16(2) (August 8, 2012):180–8.

Coughlan, K.A., Valentine, R.J., Ruderman, N.B., Saha, A.K. "Nutrient Excess in AMPK Downregulation and Insulin Resistance." *Journal of Endocrinology, Diabetes & Obesity*, 123(7) (2013):2764–72.

Saha, A.K., Balon, Xu X.J., Brandon, T.W., Kraegen, A., et al. "Insulin Resistance Due to Nutrient Excess: Is It a Consequence of AMPK Downregulation?" *Cell Cycle*, 10(20) (October 15, 2011):3447–51.

Luzzi, R., Belcaro, G., Ippolito, E. "Carotid Plaque Stabilization Induced by the Supplement Association Pycnogenol and Centella Asiatica (Centellicum)." *Minerva Cardiology and Angiology*, 64(6) (2016):603–9.

Leung, C.W., Laraia, B.A., Needham, B.L., et al. "Soda and Cell Aging: Associations Between Sugar-Sweetened Beverage Consumption and Leukocyte Telomere Length in Healthy Adults from the National Health and

Nutrition Examination Surveys." *American Journal of Public Health*, 104(12) (2014):2425–31.

Adaikalakoteswari, A., Balasubramanyam, M., Ravikumar, R., et al. "Association of Telomere Shortening with Impaired Glucose Tolerance and Diabetic Macroangiopathy." *Atherosclerosis*, 195(1) (2007):83–9.

Cheruvu, P.K., Finn, A.V., Gardner, C., et al. "Frequency and Distribution of Thin-Cap Fibroatheroma and Ruptured Plaques in Human Coronary Arteries: A Pathologic Study." *Journal of the American College of Cardiology*, 50(10) (2007):940–9.

Kolodgie, F.D., Burke, A.P., Farb, A., et al. "The Thin-Cap Fibroatheroma: A Type of Vulnerable Plaque: The Major Precursor Lesion to Acute Coronary Syndromes." *Current Opinions in Cardiology*, 16(5) (2001):285–92.

McCarthy, Christine Eileen, Yusuf, Salim, Judge, Conor, et al. "Sleep Patterns and the Risk of Acute Stroke: Results from the INTERSTROKE International Case-Control Study." *Neurology* (April 2023). https://n.neurology.org/content /neurology/early/2023/04/05/WNL.0000000000207249.full.pdf.

McDermott, Mollie, Brown, Devin L., Chervin, Ronald D. "Sleep Disorders and the Risk of Stroke." *Expert Review of Neurotherapeutics* (July 2018). https://pubmed.ncbi.nlm.nih.gov/29902391/.

Choi, MoonKi, Hayeon, Kim, Juyeon, Bae. "Does the Combination of Resistance Training and a Nutritional Intervention Have a Synergic Effect on Muscle Mass, Strength, and Physical Function in Older Adults? A Systematic Review and Meta-Analysis." *BMC Geriatrics* (November 2021). https:/ /pubmed.ncbi.nlm.nih.gov/34772342/.

Levine, Morgan E., Lu, Ake T., Quach, Austin, et al. "An Epigenetic Biomarker of Aging for Lifespan and Healthspan." *Aging* (April 2018). https:/ /www.ncbi.nlm.nih.gov/pmc/articles/PMC5940111/.

Reisman, N.R. "Anti-Aging Medicine: The Legal Issues: Legal Issues Associated with the Current and Future Practice of Anti-Aaging Medicine." *Journals of Gerontology and Biology Medical Sciences*, 59-(7) (2004):B674–B681.

Fontana, L., Meyer, T.E., Klein, S., et al. "Long-Term Calorie Restriction Is Highly Effective in Reducing the Risk for Atherosclerosis in Humans." *Proceedings of the National Academy of Science*, 101(17) (April 27, 2004):6659–63.

Most, J., Gilmore, L.A., Smith, S.R., et al. "Significant Improvement in Cardiometabolic Health in Healthy Nonobese Individuals During Caloric Restriction-Induced Weight Loss and Weight Loss Maintenance." *American Journal of Physiology-Endocrinology and Metabolism*, 314(4) (April 1, 2018):E396–E405.

Zhang, L., Zhou, G., Song, W., et al. "Pterostilbene Protects Vascular Endothelial Cells Against Oxidized Low-Density Lipoprotein-Induced Apoptosis in Vitro and in Vivo." *Apoptosis*, 17(1) (2012):25–36.

Plafki, C., Peters, P., Almeling, M., Welslau, W., Busch, R. "Complications and Side Effects of Hyperbaric Oxygen Therapy." *Aviation, Space, and Environmental Medicine*, 71 (2000);71:119–24.

Sunami, K., Takeda, Y., Hashimoto, M., Hirakawa, M. "Hyperbaric Oxygen Reduces Infarct Volume in Rats by Increasing Oxygen Supply to the Ischemic Periphery." *Critical Care Medicine*, 28 (2000):2831–36.

"Facts About Aging and Alcohol." *National Institute on Aging.* https://www.nia.nih.gov/health/facts-about-aging-and-alcohol.

Kunnumakkara, Ajaikumar B., Sailo, Bethsebie L., Banik, Kishore, et al. "Chronic Diseases, Inflammation, and Spices: How Are They Linked?" *Journal of Translational Medicine* (January 2018). https://www.ncbi.nlm.nih.gov/labs/pmc/articles/PMC5785894/.

Fatemeh, G., Sajjad, Moradi, Niloufar, Rasaei, et al. "Effect of Melatonin Supplementation on Sleep Quality: A Systematic Review and Meta-Analysis of Randomized Controlled Trials." *Journal of Neurology* (January 2022). https://pubmed.ncbi.nlm.nih.gov/33417003/.

Drouin-Chartier, Jean-Philippe, Chen, Siyu, Li, Yanping, et al. "Egg Consumption and Risk of Cardiovascular Disease: Three Large Prospective US Cohort Studies, Systematic Review, and Updated Meta-Analysis." *BMJ* (March 2020). https://www.bmj.com/content/368/bmj.m513.

Huizen, Jennifer. "All You Need to Know About Egg Yolk." *Medical News Today* (July 2023). https://www.medicalnewstoday.com/articles/320445.

Derbyshire, Emma. "Brain Health Across the Lifespan: A Systematic Review on the Role of Omega-3 Fatty Acid Supplements." *Nutrients* August 2018, https://pubmed.ncbi.nlm.nih.gov/30111738/.

Derbyshire, E. "Do Omega-3/6 Fatty Acids Have a Therapeutic Role in Children and Young People with ADHD?" *Journal of Lipids* (August 2017). https://www.ncbi.nlm.nih.gov/labs/pmc/articles/PMC5603098/.

Gordana, Petrović-Oggiano, et al. "The Effect of Walnut Consumption on n-3 Fatty Acid Profile of Healthy People Living in a Non-Mediterranean West Balkan Country, a Small Scale Randomized Study." *Nutrients* (January 2020). https://www.ncbi.nlm.nih.gov/labs/pmc/articles/PMC7019815/.

Şanlier, Nevin, et al. "Health Benefits of Fermented Foods." *Critical Reviews in Food Science and Nutrition*, National Library of Medicine, National Center for Biotechnology Information (October 2017). https://pubmed.ncbi.nlm.nih.gov /28945458/.

Zittermann, A. "Effects of Vitamin K on Calcium and Bone Metabolism." *Current Opinion in Clinical Nutrition & Metabolic Care*, 4(6) (2001):483–7.

Fry, A., Fry, A. "Vivid Dreams Explained." Sleep Foundation (December 2022). https://www.sleepfoundation.org/dreams/vivid-dreams.

Duran-Ramirez, Daniela. "Exploring the Mind-Body Connection Through Research." *Positive Psychology* (September 2020). https://positivepsychology.com/mind-body-connection/.

Esch, Tobias, Stefano, George B. "The BERN Framework of Mind-Body Medicine: Integrating Self-Care, Health Promotion, Resilience, and Applied Neuroscience." *Frontiers in Integrative Neuroscience* (July 2022).

Gilchrist, Heidi, Haynes, Abby, Olveira, Juliana S., et al. "The Value of Mind-Body Connection in Physical Activity for Older People." *Journal of Aging and Physical Activity*. https://pubmed.ncbi.nlm.nih.gov/35894992/.

Kwon, Diana. "Your Brain Could Be Controlling How Sick You Get—and How You Recover." *Nature* (February 2023). https://www.nature.com/articles/d41586-023-00509-z.

Gupta, Mayank, Sharma, Aditya. "Fear of Missing Out: A Brief Overview of Origin, Theoretical Underpinnings and Relationship with Mental Health." *World Journal of Clinical Cases* (July 2021). https://www.ncbi.nlm.nih.gov/pmc/articles/PMC8283615/.

Roelofs, Karin. "Freeze for Action: Neurobiological Mechanisms in Animal and Human Freezing." *Philosophical Transactions of the Royal Society of London B: Biological Sciences* (April 2017). https://pubmed.ncbi.nlm.nih.gov/28242739/.

Ropeik, David. "The Consequences of Fear." EMBO Reports (October 2004). https://www.ncbi.nlm.nih.gov/pmc/articles/PMC1299209/.

American Heart Association. "Recommendations for Physical Activity in Adults and Kids." Accessed 3/13/2020. https://www.heart.org/en/healthy-living/fitness/fitness-basics/aha-recs-for-physical-activity-in-adults.

"Processed Foods: What You Should Know." Mayo Clinic Health System (January 2017). www.mayoclinichealthsystem.org/hometown-health/speaking-of-health/processed-foods-what-you-should-know.

Wongcharoen, W., Jai-Aue, S. Phrommintikul, A., et al. "Effects of Curcuminoids on Frequency of Acute Myocardial Infarction After Coronary Artery Bypass Grafting." *American Journal of Cardiology,* 110(1) (2012):40–4.

Chuengsamarn, S., Rattanamongkolgul, S., Luechapudiporn, R., et al. "Curcumin Extract for Prevention of Type 2 Diabetes." *Diabetes Care,* 35(11) (2012):2121–7.

Deguchi, A. "Curcumin Targets in Inflammation and Cancer." *Endocrine, Metabolic & Immune Disorders—Drug Targets,* 15(2) (2015):88–96.

Ames, B.N. "Prevention of Mutation, Cancer, and Other Age-Associated Diseases by Optimizing Micronutrient Intake." *Journal of Nucleic Acids* (September 22, 2010).

Juanola-Falgarona, M., Salas-Salvado, J., Martinez-Gonzalez, M.A., et al. "Dietary Intake of Vitamin K Is Inversely Associated with Mortality Risk." *Journal of Nutrition*, 144(5) (May 2014):743–50.

Crichton-Stuart, Cathleen. "What Are the Benefits of Eating Healthy?" *Medical News Today* (January 2023). https://www.medicalnewstoday.com/articles/322268.

"Is Coffee Good for You or Not?" American Heart Association News (September 2018). https://www.heart.org/en/news/2018/09/28/is-coffee-good -for-you-or-not.

"Sleep Disorders and Heart Health." American Heart Association. https://www.heart.org/en/health-topics/sleep-disorders/sleep-and-heart-health.

"What Is Dementia?" Alzheimer's Association. https://www.alz.org/alzheimers-dementia/what-is-dementia.

"What Is the Mediterranean Diet?" American Heart Association, https://www.heart.org/en/healthy-living/healthy-eating/eat-smart/nutrition-basics/mediterranean-diet.

Anjum, Ibrar, Jaffery, Syeda S., Fayyaz, Muniba, et al. "The Role of Vitamin D in Brain Health: A Mini Literature Review." *Cureus* (July 2018). https://www.ncbi.nlm.nih.gov/pmc/articles/PMC6132681.

Aranow, Cynthia. "Vitamin D and the Immune System." *Journal of Investigative Medicine* (August 2011). https://www.ncbi.nlm.nih.gov/pmc/articles/PMC3166406/.

Chang, Szu-Wen, Hung-Chang, Lee. "Vitamin D and Health—the Missing Vitamin in Humans." *Pediatrics & Neonatology* (June 2019). https://pubmed.ncbi.nlm.nih.gov/31101452/.

Román, G.C., Jackson, R.E., Gadhia, R., et al. "Mediterranean Diet: The Role of Long-Chain ω-3 Fatty Acids in Fish; Polyphenols in Fruits, Vegetables, Cereals, Coffee, Tea, Cacao and Wine; Probiotics and Vitamins in Prevention of Stroke, Age-Related Cognitive Decline, and Alzheimer Disease." *Rev Neurol (Paris)* (December 2019). https://pubmed.ncbi.nlm.nih.gov/31521398/.

Shannon, Oliver M., Ranson, Janice M., Gregory, Sarah, et al. "Mediterranean Diet Adherence Is Associated with Lower Dementia Risk, Independent of Genetic Predisposition: Findings from the UK Biobank Prospective Cohort Study." *BMC Medicine* (March 2023). https://bmcmedicine.biomedcentral.com/articles/10.1186/s12916-023-02772-3.

Boege, Hedda L., et al. "Circadian Rhythms and Meal Timing: Impact on Energy Balance and Body Weight." *Current Opinion in Biotechnology* (August 2021). https://pubmed.ncbi.nlm.nih.gov/32998085/.

Davis, Rochelle, Rogers, Michelle, Coates, Alison M., et al. "The Impact of Meal Timing on Risk of Weight Gain and Development of Obesity: A Review of the Current Evidence and Opportunities for Dietary Intervention." *Current Diabetes Reports* (April 2022). https://www.ncbi.nlm.nih.gov/pmc/articles/PMC9010393/.

Logan-Sprenger, Heather M., Spriet, Lawrence L. "The Acute Effects of Fluid Intake on Urine Specific Gravity and Fluid Retention in a Mildly Dehydrated State." *Journal of Strength and Conditioning Research* (April 2013). https://pubmed.ncbi.nlm.nih.gov/22692114/.

Shirreffs, Susan M., Sawka, Michael N. "Fluid and Electrolyte Needs for Training, Competition, and Recovery." *Journal of Sports Sciences* (2011). https://pubmed.ncbi.nlm.nih.gov/22150427/.

Alcock, Joe, Maley, Carlo C., Aktipis, C. Athena. "Is Eating Behavior Manipulated by the Gastrointestinal Microbiota? Evolutionary Pressures and Potential Mechanisms." *Bioessays* (October 2014). https://www.ncbi.nlm.nih.gov/pmc/articles/PMC4270213/.

Kawano, Yoshinaga, Edwards, Madeline, Huang, Yiming, et al. "Microbiota Imbalance Induced by Dietary Sugar Disrupts Immune-Mediated Protection from Metabolic Syndrome." *Cell* (August 2022). https://doi.org/10.1016/j.cell.2022.08.005.

Jeong, Ji Na. "Effect of Pre-Meal Water Consumption on Energy Intake and Satiety in Non-Obese Young Adults." *Clinical Nutrition Research* (October 2018). https://www.ncbi.nlm.nih.gov/pmc/articles/PMC6209729/.

Moszak, Malgorzata, Szulinska, Monika, Bogdanski, Pawel. "You Are What You Eat—the Relationship Between Diet, Microbiota, and Metabolic Disorders—a Review." *Nutrients* (April 2020). https://www.ncbi.nlm.nih.gov/pmc/articles/PMC7230850/.

Cho Jeong, Hyun, Yoo, Jin Young, Kim, An Na, et al. "Association of Coffee Drinking with All-Cause and Cause-Specific Mortality in Over 190,000 Individuals: Data from Two Prospective Studies." *International Journal of Food Sciences and Nutrition* (November 2021). https://pubmed.ncbi.nlm.nih.gov/34779701/.

Gu, Xinyi, Zhang, Shuyi, Ma, Weini, et al. "The Impact of Instant Coffee and Decaffeinated Coffee on the Gut Microbiota and Depression-Like Behaviors of Sleep-Deprived Rats." *Frontiers in Microbiology* (February 2022). https://pubmed.ncbi.nlm.nih.gov/35283829/.

Gardner, Jason D., Mouton, Alan J. "Alcohol Effects on Cardiac Function." *Comprehensive Physiology* (April 2015). https://onlinelibrary.wiley.com/doi/10.1002/cphy.c140046.

Minzer, Simona, Losno, Ricardo Arturo, Casas, Rosa. "The Effect of Alcohol on Cardiovascular Risk Factors: Is There New Information?" *Nutrients* (March 2020). https://pubmed.ncbi.nlm.nih.gov/32230720/.

"The Many Ways Exercise Helps Your Heart." Harvard Health Publishing (February 2021). https://www.health.harvard.edu/heart-health/the-many-ways-exercise-helps-your-heart.

Yeap, Bu B., Marriott, J. Ross, Leen, Antonio, et al. "Serum Testosterone Is Inversely and Sex Hormone-Binding Globulin Is Directly Associated with All-Cause Mortality in Men." *Journal of Clinical Endocrinology and Metabolism* (January 2021). https://pubmed.ncbi.nlm.nih.gov/33059368/.

Kotelnicka-Gawlik, Oliwia, Skowronska, Anna, Margulska, Aleksandra, et al. "The Influence of Probiotic Supplementation on Depressive Symptoms, Inflammation, and Oxidative Stress Parameters and Fecal Microbiota in Patients with Depression Depending on Metabolic Syndrome

Comorbidity-PRO-DEMET Randomized Study Protocol." *Journal of Clinical Medicine* (March 2021). https://pubmed.ncbi.nlm.nih.gov/33804999/.

Guo, Hong, Dong, Yu-Qing, Ye, Bo-Ping. "Cranberry Extract Supplementation Exerts Preventive Effects Through Alleviating Aβ Toxicity in Caenorhabditis Elegans Model of Alzheimer's Disease." *Chinese Journal of Natural Medicines* (June 2016). https://pubmed.ncbi.nlm.nih.gov/27473960/.

Heiss, Christian, Istas, Geoffrey, Feliciano, Rodrigo P., et al. "Daily Consumption of Cranberry Improves Endothelial Function in Healthy Adults: A Double-Blind Randomized Controlled Trial." *Food & Function* (April 2022). https://pubmed.ncbi.nlm.nih.gov/35322843/.

"Anatomy of the Endocrine System." Johns Hopkins Medicine. https://www.hopkinsmedicine.org/health/wellness-and-prevention/anatomy-of-the-endocrine-system.

"Diabetes Basics." Centers for Disease Control and Prevention (October 21, 2020). https://www.cdc.gov/diabetes/basics/diabetes.html.

"The Cost of Diabetes." American Diabetes Association (October 21, 2020). https://www.diabetes.org/resources/statistics/cost-diabetes.

"Can You Reverse Sun Damage?" WebMD (August 2019). https://www.webmd.com/melanoma-skin-cancer/skin-sun-damage-treatment.

"Sun Damage." Mayo Clinic. https://www.mayoclinic.org/healthy-lifestyle/adult -health/multimedia/sun-damage/sls-20076973?s=2.

"Sun Exposure and Skin Cancer." WebMD (August 2018). https://www.webmd.com/melanoma-skin-cancer/melanoma-guide/sun-skin-cancer#1.

Amaro-Ortiz, Alexandra, Yan, Betty, D'Orazio, John A. "Ultraviolet Radiation, Aging and the Skin: Prevention of Damage by Topical cAMP Manipulation." National Center for Biotechnology Information (NCBI) (May 2015). https://www.ncbi.nlm.nih.gov/pmc/articles/PMC4344124/.

Shah, Sachin J., Oreper, Sandra, Jeon, Sun Young, et al. "Social Frailty Index: Development and Validation of an Index of Social Attributes Predictive of Mortality in Older Adults." *Proceedings of the National Academy of Sciences* (PNAS) (February 2023). https://www.pnas.org/doi/10.1073/pnas.2209414120.

Boehm, Julia K., Qureshi, Farah, Chen, Ying, et al. "Optimism and Cardiovascular Health: Longitudinal Findings from the Coronary Artery Risk Development in Young Adults Study." *Psychosomatic Medicine* (October 2020). https://pubmed.ncbi.nlm.nih.gov/32833896/.

Koga, Hayami K., Trudel-Fitzgerald, Claudia, Lee, Lewina O., et al. "Optimism, Lifestyle, and Longevity in a Racially Diverse Cohort of Women." *Journal of the American Geriatrics Society* (June 2022). https://agsjournals.onlinelibrary.wiley.com/doi/10.1111/jgs.17897.

Lee, Harold H., Kubzansky, Laura D., Okuzono, Sakurako S., et al. "Optimism and Risk of Mortality Among African-Americans: The Jackson Heart Study." *Preventive Medicine* (January 2022). https://pubmed.ncbi.nlm.nih.gov/34863812/.

Burgess, Lana. "12 Foods to Boost Brain Function." *Medical News Today* (January 2020). https://www.medicalnewstoday.com/articles/324044.

Gardener, Samantha L., Rainey-Smith, Stephanie R. "The Role of Nutrition in Cognitive Function and Brain Ageing in the Elderly." *Current Nutrition Reports* (September 2018). https://pubmed.ncbi.nlm.nih.gov/29974344/.

Hale, M. Jo et al. "Does Postponing Retirement Affect Cognitive Function? A Counterfactual Experiment to Disentangle Life Course Risk Factors." *SSM-Population Health* (September 2021).

Xue, Baowen, Cadar, Dorina, Fleishmann, Maria, et al. "Effect of Retirement on Cognitive Function: The Whitehall II Cohort Study." *European Journal of Epidemiology* (December 2017).

Index

Acknowledgments

I am grateful to God for my amazing parents, who taught me hard work, perseverance, and determination to have an influence in people's lives. To Valerie Borchardt, my agent, I am forever grateful. You believed in me from day one.

Lorraine Zenka was an enormous help in this massive undertaking. Her experience as an editor makes me proud of the result. Whenever I got overwhelmed, Lorraine was there to help and offer brilliant suggestions to help me go on. Lorraine, I know I would not have completed this book without you. Thanks to you, I am immensely proud of the end result.

I have so many more people to thank, including Dina Cheney, who contributed her fantastic recipes. The author of six cookbooks, her delicious recipes provide not only health benefits but are nothing short of true perfection. I also want to thank Melba Wilson and the editors at Kevin Anderson & Associates. I would like to thank Christine Belleris, Lindsey Triebel, and Christian Blonshine for believing in *The Ageless Revolution* and the importance of getting the word out.

I am also grateful to my publicist, Sandi Mendelson.

Finally, I owe it all to my patients. I am grateful for *your* expressions of gratitude as you triumphed over severe diseases without using drugs. Your significant improvements in overall health are, undoubtedly, my life's greatest accomplishments.

About the Author

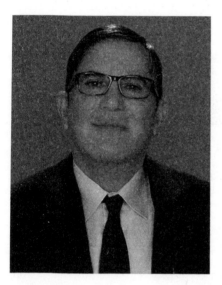

Michael Aziz is a physician, author, and broadcast media commentator. He is board certified in internal medicine and an attending physician at Lenox Hill Hospital in New York City. He also maintains a private practice in Manhattan and the Hamptons. Dr. Aziz completed his training at Long Island Jewish Medical Center and Staten Island University Hospital in New York. Dr. Aziz is a member of the American College of Physicians and the American Society of Internal Medicine. He is also a fellow of the Royal Society of Medicine in the United Kingdom.

Dr. Aziz has appeared as a keynote speaker before many prestigious groups nationally and internationally, including the American Academy of Anti-Aging Medicine. Dr. Aziz has his own private practice that focuses on functional medicine and modern advances in the medical field. In his bestselling first book, *The Perfect 10 Diet*, Dr. Aziz demonstrated the danger of low-fat diets and synthetic hormones. This fueled his concentration on anti-aging, natural remedies, supplements, peptides, bioidentical hormones,

and a natural diet. The practical application of all these innovations became the foundation of *The Ageless Revolution*.

Dr. Aziz wrote for *Bottomline Newsletters*, which provided health advice to millions of readers. He also writes the "Ask the Doctor" column for *Life Extension* magazine. Dr. Aziz's columns, articles, and opinions have been published in the *Los Angeles Times*, CNN, WebMD, *New York Post*, the *New York Daily News*, the *Washington Post*, and in many national and international magazines. Dr. Aziz has done medical commentary on many networks, including NPR, *Fox and Friends*, ABC, WGN Chicago, NBC, and Telemundo.

Dr. Aziz is also passionate about volunteerism and philanthropy. He volunteered at clinics for the uninsured in New York City for two years after his residency. In 2018, he volunteered in rural areas of Indonesia, managing all of the patients' medical needs. During the Covid-19 pandemic, he raised funds for much-needed personal protection equipment for his hospital staff in New York City.

Scan the QR code for *The Ageless Revolution* website.